Understanding Your Changing Life

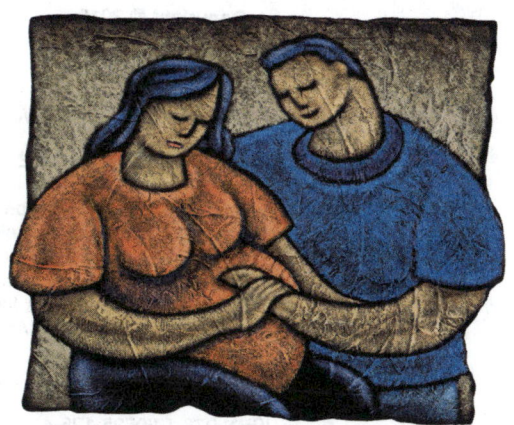

Linda G. Smock
Principal, Gulf Coast Christian School
St. Petersburg, Florida
Former Supervisor, Family and Consumer Sciences and Health Science Education
Pinellas County Schools, Pinellas County, Florida

Publisher
The Goodheart-Willcox Company, Inc.
Tinley Park, Illinois

Copyright © 2010

by

The Goodheart-Willcox Company, Inc.

Previous edition copyright 2002

All rights reserved. No part of this work may be reproduced, stored, or transmitted in any form or by any electronic or mechanical means, including information storage and retrieval systems, without the prior written permission of The Goodheart-Willcox Company, Inc. Manufactured in the United States of America.

Library of Congress Catalog Card Number 2008051975

ISBN 978-1-60525-126-4

1 2 3 4 5 6 7 8 9 – 10 – 14 13 12 11 10 09

Library of Congress Cataloging-in-Publication Data

Smock, Linda G.
  Understanding your changing life / Linda G. Smock.
    p. cm.
Includes index.
ISBN 978-1-60525-126-4
  1. Teenage mothers. 2. Motherhood. 3. Infants--Care. 4. Teenage pregnancy. I. Title.
  RG 556.5.S664 2010
  649'.10242--dc22

2008051975

About the Author

Linda G. Smock has taught Family Living and Child Development classes for middle school, high school, and college students and has worked with many pregnant students. Currently, Linda serves as principal of Gulf Coast Christian School in St. Petersburg, Florida.

Formerly, she held the position of supervisor of Family and Consumer Sciences and Health Science Education in Pinellas County, Florida. For 20 years, Linda served as facilitator of the Pinellas County Family Life Education Committee, working to help teens and concerned citizens in the community reach a consensus on sexuality education issues.

Linda is active in the community and dedicated to helping youth make important decisions for building solid foundations in their lives. She has served on advisory boards for health-related agencies and on the board of trustees for a private school.

Acknowledgments

We would like to thank the following professionals who reviewed the original text and provided valuable input:

Cathy Allison
GRADS Coordinator
Auburn Career Center
Concord, Ohio

Dawn Gale Aspacher
Parent Educator
Child and Family Resources, Inc.
The Center for
   Adolescent Parents
Tucson, Arizona

JoAnn J. Bartek
FCS Teacher/Director,
   Student Parent Team SCLC
Lincoln High School
Lincoln, Nebraska

Martha Hamdani-Swain
former Program Coordinator,
Pregnancy Education
   and Parenting Program
Jack Yates High School
Houston, Texas

Sheree M. Moser
FCS Department Chair
   and District Assistant
Lincoln High School
Lincoln, Nebraska

Sara McDonald Rohar
Project Director, Young Mother's
   Program
Birmingham City Schools
Birmingham, Alabama

Carol J. Sullivan, RN
Chairman, New Mexico GRADS
   Curriculum Committee
Socorro, New Mexico

Table of Contents

Part One
Understanding Yourself

Chapter 1
Pregnancy: A Life-Changing Event 14

- Handling the News 15
- Accepting the Situation 15
  - Which Things Will Change? 16
  - Which Things Will Stay the Same? 23
- Telling Others About the Pregnancy 24
  - Choosing the Right Time 24
  - Choosing the Right Way 25
  - Handling Negative Reactions 26
- Preparing to Make a Decision 28
- The Skills You Will Need to Succeed 28
  - Making Decisions 28
  - Building Relationships 29
  - Meeting Your Child's Needs 31
  - Coping in the Outside World 32

Chapter 2
Improving Your Self-Esteem 34

- What Is Self-Esteem? 34
- Why Is Self-Esteem Important? 35
  - Personal Outlook 35
  - Health and Personal Care 36

Goals and Performance 36
　　　Decision Making 37
　　　Relationships 38
　　　Parenting 38
　How Is Self-Esteem Formed? 39
　Evaluating Your Self-Esteem 42
　How Can You Improve Your Self-Esteem? 43
　　　Get to Know Yourself 43
　　　Use Positive Self-Talk 43
　　　Learn to Visualize Success 46
　　　Talk with a Professional 46
　　　Strengthen Your Support System 47
　　　Take Responsibility for Your Life 48

Chapter 3
Considering Values, Goals, and Decisions 50
　Values 50
　　　How Are Values Developed? 51
　　　Value Conflicts 55
　　　How Are Values Changed? 56
　Goals and Resources 57
　　　Goals Are Often Based on Values 58
　　　Resources Help You Reach Goals 58
　　　You Can Learn How to Set Goals 60
　Decision Making 62
　　　Identify the Decision to Be Made 62
　　　Gather and Examine Information 63
　　　Identify Your Options 65
　　　Evaluate Each Option 65
　　　Choose the Best Option and Act on It 66
　　　Evaluate the Results of Your Decision 67

Chapter 4
Is Marriage in the Picture? 69

    What Is Love? 69
    Other Reasons Teens Marry 71
        Pregnancy 71
        To Cure Loneliness 72
        To Make Them Feel Complete 73
        To Escape Unhappy Home Lives 74
        To Gain Money or Social Status 75
        To Become Life Partners 75
    Why Do Some Teen Marriages Fail? 76
    How Are Marital Roles Changing? 78
    How Do Couples Adjust to Marriage? 79
    Examining Your Situation 80
        Is Marriage an Option Right Now? 81
        Is This the Right Person for You? 82
        Are You Ready to Marry? 84
        What About Waiting? 85

Chapter 5
What Does It Mean to Be a Parent? 89

    Parenting Responsibilities and Rewards 90
    To Parent or Not to Parent? 91
        Factors to Consider 93
    Am I Ready to Be a Parent? 96
    Parenting Options for Teens 97
        Within a Marriage 98
        As Co-Parents 99
        With the Support of Family 100
        On Your Own 102

Chapter 6
An Important Decision 105
- Parenting 105
- Adoption 107
  - Adoption Agencies 108
  - Independent Adoption 110
  - Openness in Adoption 112
  - Reasons for Choosing Adoption 113
  - The Adoption Process 114
  - Feelings About Adoption 114
- Abortion 116
  - Medical Issues 117
  - Emotional and Social Issues 118
- Thinking Through the Decision 120
  - Identify the Decision to Be Made 120
  - Gather and Examine Information 120
  - Identify Your Options 121
  - Evaluate Each Option 121
  - Choose the Best Option and Act on It 122
  - Evaluate the Result of Your Decision 122

Part Two
Your Changing Relationships

Chapter 7
Adjusting to Life as a Teen Parent 126
- Comparing the Roles of Teen and Parent 126
- Adjustments a Baby Demands 128
  - Managing Your Time 129
  - Managing Your Money 131
  - Managing Your Schoolwork 133
  - Keeping a Part-Time Job 135
  - Finding a Good Babysitter 137
- Changing Expectations in Your Relationships 138
  - With Your Family 139
  - With Your Co-Parent 142
  - With Your Partner 146
  - With Your Friends 147

Dealing with Stress 149
    Causes of Stress for Teen Parents 149
    Effects of Stress 151
    Ways to Reduce Stress 153
    Ways to Prevent Stress 154

Chapter 8
Relationships and Sexual Decision Making 156

Building a Healthy Relationship 156
    Recognizing an Unhealthy Relationship 158
Making Responsible Sexual Decisions 160
    Factors to Consider 162
    Choosing Abstinence 166
Preventing Sexually Transmitted Infections 167
    HIV/AIDS 169
    Chlamydia 170
    Gonorrhea 170
    Genital Herpes 171
    Genital Warts 172
    Syphilis 172
    Hepatitis Type B 173
    Trichomoniasis 174
    Pubic Lice 175
    Scabies 176
    Vaginal Infections 176
    What to Do If You Think You Have an STI 176
Preventing a Repeat Pregnancy 178
    Contraceptive Methods 180
    Deciding About Contraception 188

Chapter 9
Communicating for Better Relationships 190

Key Elements of Communication 191
    Types of Communication 191
    Active Listening 192
    Effective Speaking 196
    Learning to Handle Anger 198
    Being Assertive 199
Barriers to Good Communication 201

Communicating with Others 203
- Children 203
- Co-Parent 204
- Parents 206

Conflict Resolution 207
- Causes of Conflict 207
- Conflict Outcomes 208
- Ways to Handle Conflict 208
- Steps in Conflict Resolution 209

Chapter 10
Crises in Relationships 213

Common Crises for Teens 214
- Depression 215
- Domestic Violence 219
- Sexual Assault, Rape, and Incest 226
- Substance Abuse and Addictions 231

Responding to Crises 233
- Personal Resources 233
- Family Influences 235
- Community Resources 237
- Nonhuman Resources 240

Glossary 241

Index 250

Transitions:
A Series for Pregnant and Parenting Teens

Understanding Your Changing Life
by Linda G. Smock

This two-part book addresses the transitions teen pregnancy and parenting bring. Topics include: self-esteem; values, goals, options, and decisions related to pregnancy; adjusting to parenthood; communication; relationships with family, friends and co-parent; partner relationships and sexual decisions; birth control; STIs; and crises in relationships.

Your New Baby
by Angela M. Nicoletti, RNC, WHNP

By telling teens what to expect, this book reduces the fear and mystery of pregnancy and childbirth. Topics include: prenatal development; eating, exercise, and health care recommendations; preparations for parenting; labor and delivery; the postpartum period; and newborn care.

Helping Your Child Grow and Develop
by Karen Zimmerman, Ph.D.

This book suggests practical ways for teen parents to promote development; identify and meet a child's needs; provide a safe, loving environment; guide behavior; and choose quality child care. Developmental Milestones charts describe each area of development for infants and toddlers.

Building Your Future
by Sally R. Campbell

This book helps teen parents learn to manage their lives, their families, and their futures. It explains how to find help, handle legal issues, manage money and resources; shop wisely; use credit and financial accounts; set goals, and become a successful worker.

Introduction

When you learn you're involved in a pregnancy, you will experience many emotions at once. This is a major transition in your life! After the initial shock wears off, reality will hit. You'll start to think about all the decisions that lie ahead. These choices can be tough to make, but you can do it. Reading this book can help.

<u>Understanding Your Changing Life</u> addresses many of the changes you will face as a result of teen pregnancy and parenting. Part One will help you understand the issues related to teen pregnancy and guide you through the decision-making process. Topics include the following:

- telling others
- improving your self-esteem
- considering your values, goals, and decisions
- marriage, parenting, adoption, and abortion
- deciding which option is right for you

Part Two focuses on adjustments you will make and changes you can expect in your life and relationships if you parent. Topics include adjusting to teen parenting; healthy relationships; making responsible sexual decisions; preventing STIs and repeat pregnancies; communication; and crises within relationships.

Much of the language in this book is directed to females, because they will experience the physical changes of pregnancy and childbirth. However, a young man who is involved in a pregnancy can gain much from reading this book, too. His support and involvement are very important to his partner, their baby, and himself.

Your baby may be a girl or a boy. To make the chapters easier to read, we have referred to your baby in some sections as <u>he</u> and in other sections as <u>she</u>. We hope this will also help you relate to the chapters in a personal way as you think about your baby.

Part One
Understanding Yourself

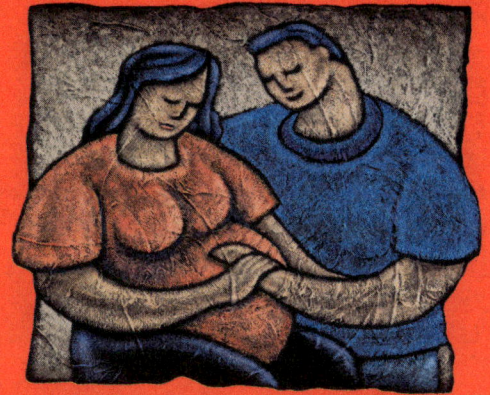

"It won't happen to me," but sometimes it does. Teen pregnancy brings many serious questions with no easy answers. Only after taking a look deep inside yourself will you find the answers you seek. The first six chapters of this book will help you do just that by

♣ offering an honest look at what lies ahead,

♣ helping you evaluate your self-esteem,

♣ guiding you to explore your values and goals,

♣ emphasizing responsible, step-by-step decision making, and

♣ presenting your options in an informative, unbiased way.

Chapter 1
Pregnancy:
A Life-Changing
Event

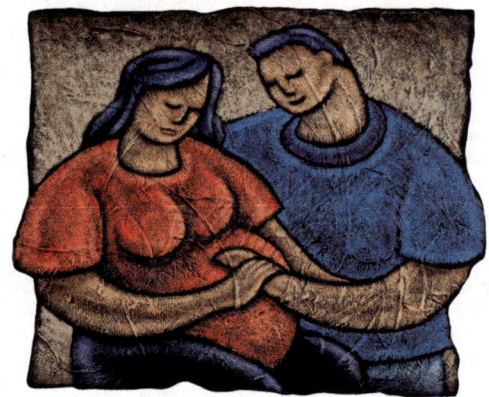

You may have just learned you or your partner is pregnant. You may feel this pregnancy is the end of the world. In fact, it's just the beginning of a new world you will experience. You may be wondering what will happen now. The challenges you face will not be easy. You may be having mixed feelings—torn between wanting to parent and wanting to be "just a normal teen." Some days you may resent the pregnancy. At other times, you may find joy in the changes pregnancy brings. If you have these conflicting feelings, you're not alone. This is a normal part of teen pregnancy.

This is the first chapter in a series of books that will help guide you through decisions regarding pregnancy and your life. In this chapter, you will learn how important it is to accept your situation and move on with your life. Although the news can be shocking, your life will continue. You have much to decide and do. This chapter also describes some of the skills you will need to succeed. These skills relate to the tasks that lie ahead of you as a pregnant teen or the partner of a pregnant teen.

If you're the soon-to-be father, this series of books is for you, too. You may notice that, for clarity's sake, much of the wording is directed to young women who are pregnant. However, most of the topics also apply to you. You may have some additional concerns. Find someone who can help you think things through and talk about your concerns. If at all possible, it's good for you to participate in the decisions related to the pregnancy. You and your partner (or former partner) created the pregnancy together. Both of you should be involved in deciding what to do next.

Handling the News

When you find out you're pregnant, you may feel overwhelmed with emotion. At first, you may feel numb. You may not believe it's real. Some teens question the results of the pregnancy test. You may decide to have another test done just to be sure. When the results are the same, you may feel a mixture of shock, anger, sadness, fear, and guilt. In addition to these difficult feelings, you may also feel joy and happiness. These feelings are normal.

In the first few days after the test, you may go back and forth between all these feelings. You will probably keep repeating to yourself, "I'm pregnant." It may seem like the entire situation is just a dream, even though you know it's real. See Figure 1-1. Many thoughts and unanswered questions may race through your mind about what lies ahead. Be patient—you will work through all this in time.

Some teens feel depressed when they learn they're pregnant. If you have thoughts of hurting yourself, seek help. Suicide is not an answer to your problems. All that would do is end your life. You have much to offer—the world needs you. Ending your life would also be devastating for your friends and family. You can work through the problems created by your pregnancy and find a better solution.

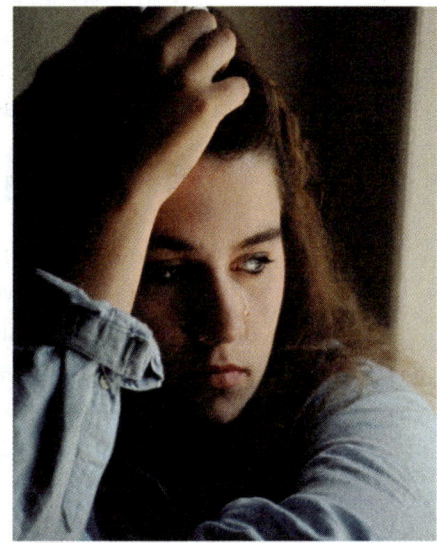

1-1 When you first learn of your pregnancy, you may have mixed feelings. You may not even believe all this is really happening to you.

Find someone who will listen to your concerns. Talk to your parents or a health care provider, teacher, school nurse, or counselor. Trusted friends and relatives are also an option. You might be able to call a pregnancy helpline, teen talkline, or crisis hot line. Many of these services answer calls 24 hours a day. Look in the phone book for hot line numbers in your area.

Accepting the Situation

Once the initial shock wears off, it's time to start sorting things out. You need to accept this situation and move on with your life.

Sometimes this can be hard to do. It can be hard to believe you're really pregnant, especially when you're not showing yet and you can't feel the baby move.

Ignoring your pregnancy will not make it go away. Some pregnant teens pretend they're not really pregnant. They delay seeking medical care and making important decisions. In the long run, this hurts both them and their babies. Deal with things as they really are. This will allow you to make decisions about what's best for you.

As a result of the pregnancy, many things will change. This experience will change your life. Even in the midst of all these changes, some things about your life will stay the same. Knowing more about what lies ahead can prepare you to accept the changes and move on with your life.

Which Things Will Change?

In the early months of your pregnancy, you will likely spend lots of time thinking. You will be trying to imagine how your life is going to change. Much of this thinking may focus on reality. You'll probably spend time daydreaming and fantasizing, too. This is normal. You're trying to make this new situation (pregnancy) fit into your understanding of your life. It takes some time to blend the two together. Identifying the changes ahead is the first step in planning how you will deal with them.

Physical and Emotional Changes

In pregnancy, many changes take place within your body. Your emotions may change quickly, too. Some of these changes are minor, while others may bother you more. It can help to learn more about the normal physical and emotional changes of pregnancy. This can reassure you about what's happening to you. It can also alert you if there's a problem. (Another book in this series called <u>Your New Baby</u> describes these changes in more detail.)

Seek Medical Care. You need to seek medical care as soon as you think you might be pregnant. This care can protect your health and the health of your unborn child. The medical care given in pregnancy is called prenatal care. (Prenatal means before birth.) You can get this care from a health care provider at a health department, clinic, or private practice. See Figure 1-2.

This type of medical care includes tests to check your health and your baby's health. Your health care provider will monitor your pregnancy and be sure all is going well. He or she can treat any problems that arise. This can lessen the chance a problem will become more serious. Your provider will also advise you on how to take care of yourself while you're pregnant.

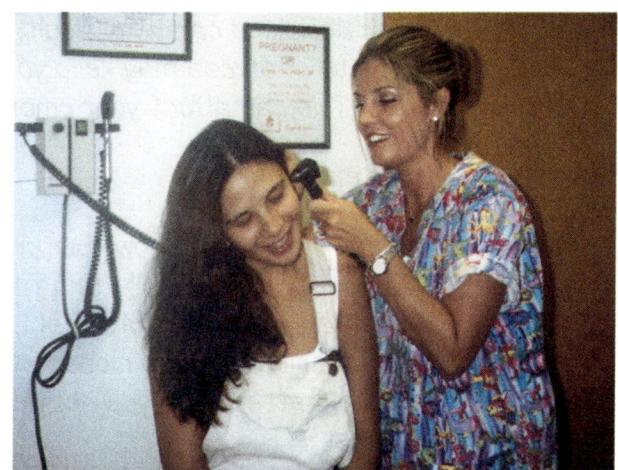

1-2 Seeking quality health care throughout your pregnancy will increase your chances of having a healthy baby.

Some of the changes in your body will cause you discomfort. Dealing with these changes is a big part of adjusting to early pregnancy. As the pregnancy progresses, most of these discomforts will pass and others will begin. Each person will experience these problems differently.

Even if you're not sure what you will do about your pregnancy, it's best to have prenatal care. That way, you and your baby will be as healthy as possible no matter what you decide. Prenatal care makes it less likely your baby will be born too early or too small. Babies born too early or too small often have serious health problems.

An Emotional Roller Coaster. To support a growing baby, your body needs to make some changes. Your hormones control and direct these changes. (A *hormone* is a chemical that controls or affects one of your body systems.) Changing hormone levels may affect your moods. For instance, you might cry for no reason or get quite angry over a minor problem.

Adjusting to your situation may also cause emotional changes and mood swings. You have a lot to think about and handle. You may have mixed feelings about the pregnancy or what you will do now.

These decisions can be difficult, and they can create stress. High amounts of stress may keep you from responding as you normally would. This can affect your emotions, too.

Relationships

You may wonder how your pregnancy will affect your relationships with your partner, family, and friends. Each situation is unique. You can be sure these relationships will change, though. Some relationships will grow closer, while others may have problems. This is true no matter what you decide to do regarding the pregnancy.

Learning you're pregnant may change how you feel about these relationships. A relationship may seem more or less important to you in light of the changes you're facing. When you share the news with someone, his or her reaction may also change the relationship.

Partner. When you find out you're pregnant, you may think about how this will change your relationship with your partner. It depends on many factors. First, what was the relationship like just before you learned of the pregnancy? Were you still together? Was the relationship close or casual? Was it new or long-lasting? Was it respectful or unhealthy? The answers to these questions will tell you much about the changes ahead.

When your partner learns of the pregnancy, this can change the relationship. Much depends on his reaction to the news. See Figure 1-3. Will he stay by your side throughout the pregnancy? Will you stay together and maybe even consider marriage? On the other hand, will he end the relationship and refuse to speak to you again? Either reaction is possible. You can see how these responses can send a relationship in opposite directions.

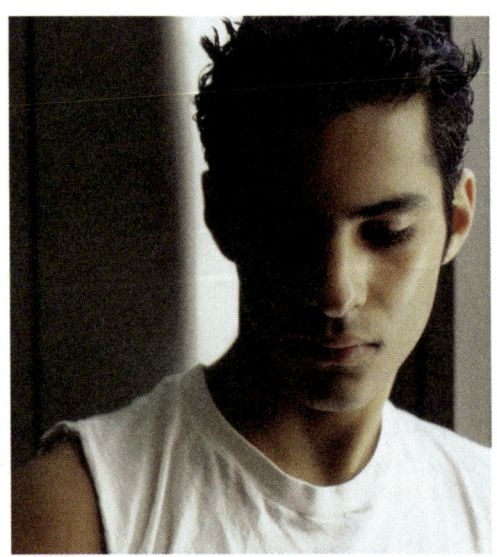

1-3 Like you, your partner may have mixed feelings about your pregnancy. Give him some time to think things through.

Family. Most families have a strong reaction to the news their teen is pregnant or caused a pregnancy. It often comes as a shock. Parents may feel overwhelmed with emotion. They probably wanted other things for your life. Your parents may be thinking of how hard it must be in your position. When you're hurting, they hurt, too. Parents also have their own feelings of disappointment, disbelief, grief, anger, and sadness. Some parents may be excited and happy about becoming grandparents.

A parent's initial reaction may or may not reflect how the relationship will be in the future. After your parent has had time to adjust to the news, he or she may be quite supportive. Many teens in this situation find a parent is their best support. They turn to their parents for guidance and understanding. For others, the relationship with their parents is more of a struggle. The quality of the relationship before the pregnancy often predicts how it will be in the future.

How your parents respond may also depend on what you plan to do regarding the pregnancy. If your parents don't agree with your decisions, they may express disapproval and be quite upset with you. This can be hard to take, especially if you believe you're making the right choices. Talk to them about how you feel, but realize you may not be able to change their views.

Friends. Now that you're pregnant (or your partner is), you may place a different value on some of the friendships you had before. It may seem like you can't relate to your friends' concerns and they can't relate to yours. You may see yourself growing up faster than they are because of all you're dealing with. As a result, some of these friendships may drift apart.

You may also have some friends who don't respond well to the news of the pregnancy. They may not want to be friends anymore. These people may not feel comfortable around you because they can't relate to your situation. This can be painful, but you can find the strength to accept these changes and move on with your life.

On the other hand, you may find some of your friends are quite supportive. These are true friends who really care about you as a person. You can talk to them about what is going on in your life. They will respect your decisions and stand by you. Still other people who were not close to you before the pregnancy will step forward and become your friends. These new friends can be good ones, too.

Plans, Goals, and Dreams

You may think a great deal about how your plans, goals, and dreams will be affected by the pregnancy. Some of these plans may seem minor. Suppose you had planned to take a class trip for spring break. With all that's going on, you may not be able to go. You may feel disappointed about this. Larger goals, such as graduating from high school, will have a bigger impact on your life. Think about how pregnancy will alter these goals.

It may seem you're missing out on a lot of things because of the pregnancy. You're probably gaining some new experiences, also. You can still find ways to meet many of your goals. It may take some extra time, patience, and creativity, but you can do it. (You can learn more about career and educational goals in another title in this series, <u>Building Your Future</u>.)

School. When you find out about your pregnancy, one of your biggest fears may be facing people at school. You may wonder what they will think and how they will treat you. You may worry about feeling different from the other students.

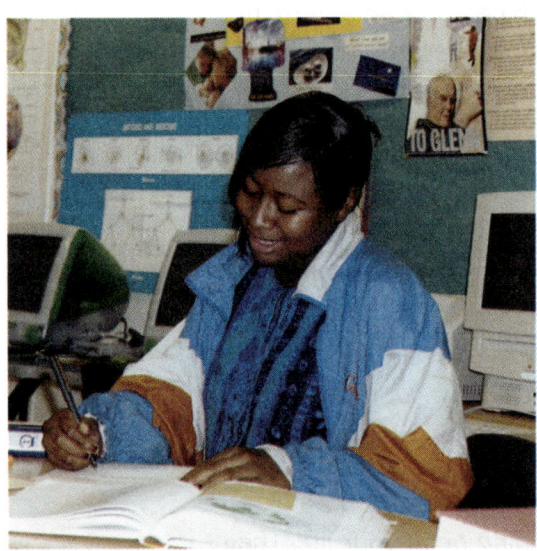

1-4 Although concentrating on schoolwork can be hard right now, it's important to your future.

The reactions of others <u>can</u> be hard to handle. Think about how you'll answer questions that seem too personal. Remember you don't have to tell people any more than you want about your life. Having some responses prepared can make this easier. Feel confident you will make the best decision for your life. You don't have to justify this with anyone. Try your best not to let other people and their reactions bother you too much.

Finishing your education is crucial to your future. See Figure 1-4. This will allow you to qualify for decent-paying jobs in the future. You will need a job that can support you (and your child if you decide to parent). Graduating may be a necessary step toward meeting your career goals. For these reasons, you need to try to stay in school even when things get tough.

It may be harder for a young woman to attend school while she's pregnant. She may have some physical discomforts that make it more difficult. Nausea and fatigue can make it hard to concentrate. She will probably spend a lot of time in the restroom. This can be annoying, especially when it interrupts class. Later in pregnancy, it may be hard to get comfortable in school desks as her abdomen grows.

The realities of the situation may also make it hard to concentrate. You have a lot on your mind right now. All that's going on in your life right now may seem to matter much more than classroom lectures and homework. It's important to do your best, however. Finding someone to talk to about your concerns may make it easier to focus during the school day.

If you continue your pregnancy, you'll need to talk to school personnel about your situation. It might help to take a parent or trusted adult with you. Work with your teachers, counselor, and nurse. In some schools, you may also need to talk to your principal about your plans. Let the school personnel know what your needs are. For instance, you'll miss some school when your baby is born. Develop a plan for making up this work. Your teachers and counselor can help you finish school successfully. If these people are not helpful, talk to your parents or a trusted adult.

You may need to adjust your school schedule. Ask your health care provider if you can keep going to physical education classes and sports practices. Make sure none of your class activities will expose you to harmful chemicals. If you're very tired, you may need to drop some of your after-school activities, too. You don't want to push yourself too hard at this time.

Work. If you have a part-time job, you may wonder how pregnancy will affect your ability to keep working. This depends on the kind of job you have and how your pregnancy goes. If you didn't have a job before, you may wonder if it's safe to start one. Making some extra money right now might be really helpful.

In either case, safety is your first concern. Is the job you're doing (or considering) safe for a pregnant woman? See Figure 1-5 for questions about job safety during pregnancy. You should also talk to your health care provider. He or she can tell you whether the job you've chosen is safe. If it's a risky job for you or your baby now, think about taking another, safer job.

You will also want to think about your ability to perform the job. Will pregnancy keep you from meeting any of your job duties? In most cases, it won't. If you have concerns about your job duties, talk to your employer. He or she might have ideas about ways you could change your job duties for now.

Working may be harder while you're pregnant. This is true for many of the same reasons attending school can be harder now. Nausea and frequent urination can make it hard to focus on your job. Emotional concerns can affect your concentration, too. Fatigue can make working harder. Before you were pregnant, it may have been easy to combine school and work. Now keeping this schedule may be more difficult. Getting enough rest is important. Keep this in mind as you make decisions about working.

Is This Job Safe for Me?

Safety is your first consideration when it comes to working while you're pregnant. Ask yourself the following questions about the job you have or one you're considering:

* Does this job expose me to lots of people with various illnesses and infections? This is typical of jobs in the medical field or those that involve working with children. You want to protect yourself and your baby from these illnesses and infections.
* Does this job expose me to radiation, lead, or dangerous chemicals? Avoid these substances because they can harm your unborn child.
* Does my job require me to lift heavy loads or operate dangerous machinery? Heavy lifting is not safe during pregnancy. Since you'll be feeling more tired than usual, it may not be a good idea to operate dangerous machinery, either.
* Do I have to stand for long periods of time? If so, can I take breaks often to sit down and put my feet up? This can reduce swelling and increase circulation.
* Do I have to sit for long periods of time? If so, can I get up and walk around every hour or so?

1-5 Use these questions to determine if the job you have (or are considering) is safe during pregnancy.

Other Changes. School and work are not the only areas in which your plans, goals, and dreams will change. Other areas of your personal life will also be affected by your pregnancy. The biggest change may be in how you spend your free time. You may have spent a great deal of time with your friends. Your priorities may change as a result of the pregnancy. While you're busy making plans about the pregnancy, you may need to spend more time alone.

If you will be parenting, the way you spend your money will be changing. Now you have someone else to think about. You probably won't be able to spend much money on yourself for items you don't really need. If you have to pay prenatal care costs, these can be expensive. Buying baby supplies and maternity clothes can take a lot of money, too. Starting a savings account now is also a good idea. This can help with some of your expenses after the baby is born.

Which Things Will Stay the Same?

When thinking of all these changes, you may feel overwhelmed. It may seem like your whole life has been turned upside down. Not everything has changed, however. Some things are still the same. Remembering these things can help you feel stable in the midst of uncertainty.

Most importantly, you are still the same person you were before the pregnancy. You still have the same strengths (and weaknesses). These parts of you haven't changed. You won't lose the skills, abilities, and talents you had before, either. Becoming pregnant doesn't take these things away from you. It doesn't make you a bad person or a failure. See Figure 1-6.

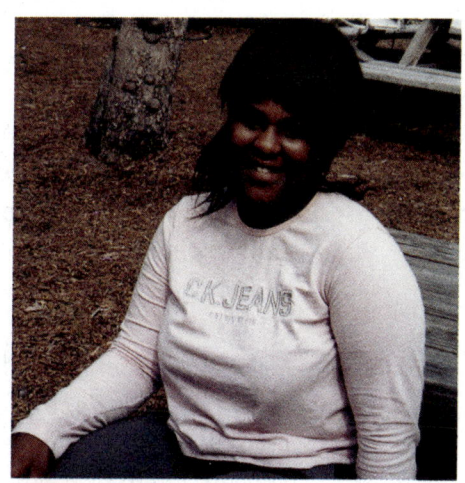

1-6 Pregnancy changes much about your life, but it doesn't change the person you are inside.

Can you think of other things that won't change because of pregnancy? At first, you have to adjust to pregnancy. As things start to settle down, you may notice less has changed than you had first thought. For instance, once you've adjusted, your school day may be much the same as always. You'll have the same classes, assignments, and teachers.

Telling Others About the Pregnancy

You may think a lot about what you will tell others about your pregnancy. You may wonder whom to tell and when to tell them. It can be hard to know how to handle this. You may be tempted not to tell anyone. This is not wise. At this time, you really need the support of someone close to you. Going through this alone can make it harder than it already is.

On the other hand, you also don't need to tell everyone you know just yet. You may want to share this news with just a few important people. This is especially true if you're still deciding what to do regarding the pregnancy.

Start by telling someone you know will be supportive. This person will listen to you and not say things that will hurt your feelings. He or she will help you think things through. This person can help you decide when and how to tell others.

Choosing the Right Time

Pick the best time to tell others about your pregnancy. This will make sharing the news a little easier. It will also help ensure you will get the best possible response to your news. You will want to tell some people before others, but make sure the timing feels right for each one.

Most teens feel the need to tell their parents fairly soon. This way they can "get it over with" and not have to keep dreading their parents' response. Telling your parents is also usually better than having them find out on their own. Your parents may soon notice when your pregnancy starts to show. Hiding your pregnancy from them is probably not a good idea. This might keep you from getting the prenatal care and support you need.

When you're ready to tell your parents, timing is still important. You know your parents well. When is the best time of day to have a serious conversation with them? Choose the time when they're most likely to be relaxed and available to you. If you know your parents are having a really bad day, you might wait a day or so to tell them. They may respond with more compassion when they're in a better mood. If their bad mood seems to last several days, you may need to tell them anyway. You don't want to delay too long.

You should probably also tell your partner soon. He's involved in the pregnancy, too. You'll want to know what he has to say. His response may influence your decisions. If you have serious concerns about telling him, talk with a trusted adult. In a few cases, it might be safer not to tell him.

The next people you tell might be a few close friends. These people care about you as a person and will support you. See Figure 1-7. Share the news with these friends when you feel ready. You might have a friend who is likely to share your news with others. Wait to tell this person until it doesn't matter to you if he or she tells someone else.

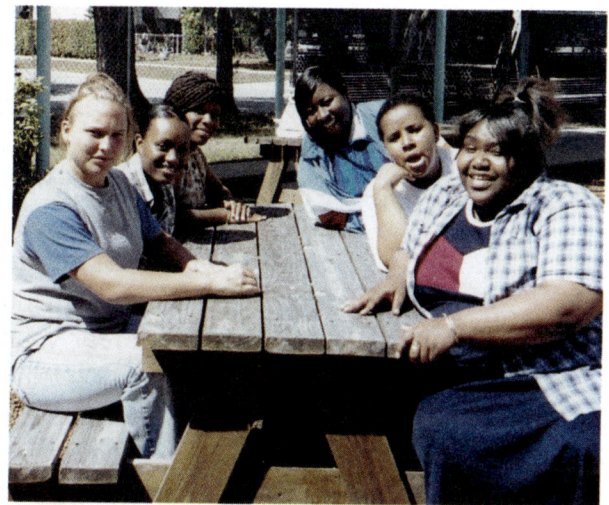

1-7 A strong network of friends can be a great support to you in this time of change.

You may want to wait a while before telling most other people. When you know what you will do regarding the pregnancy, you can choose whether to tell them and what to say. This can also help other people respond in a way that's helpful for you. Imagine how you would feel if a friend brought you a bunch of baby clothes because she didn't know you were planning an adoption for your child. That might be hard for you, which is one reason choosing the right time is important.

Choosing the Right Way

For each person you will tell, think about how you will share the news. Think about how to word your message. The words you choose may affect how the person responds. What do you want to tell this person? What would you rather not discuss? Deciding this ahead of time helps you share only what you want.

Just as important as what you will say is how you will say it. Think about the person you're telling. How do you expect he or she will respond? This might influence the way you choose to share the news. You have a few options. These include the following:

- sharing a private conversation
- giving the news over the phone
- having a trusted adult with you during the discussion
- writing a letter
- having someone else tell the person for you

Talking in private works well when you expect the person to be calm and supportive. When you know he or she will be happy for you, this can be the most fun way to share the news. If the person lives far away, a phone call may be your best option. You may not prefer this method for someone who lives close, though.

Sometimes it's best to have help from a trusted adult. Suppose you fear your parents might hurt you or ask you to leave home. This might also help if you fear your partner's reaction will be explosive. Ask this trusted adult to join you in telling, or ask him or her to do it for you. This might make the initial reaction safer for you.

Writing a letter can also be a good option. This lets you say everything you want to say without being interrupted. It allows the other person to have an initial reaction without involving you. A person might respond to you better when he or she has had time to think about the situation.

You know the people in your life best. If you think about their personalities, you can choose the best way to share the news. This will help things go more smoothly. It may help reduce the stress of telling people about the pregnancy.

Handling Negative Reactions

Of course you want all the people you tell about your pregnancy to respond in a warm and supportive way. If this happens, you'll be very lucky. When a woman shares this news with others, she may find not everyone is thrilled. Her friends and family may be concerned about how things will work out. They may think she's making a wrong decision.

Pregnant teens often receive more negative reactions than adult women do. Teen pregnancy often brings with it many challenges. People don't always respond as well as you'd like. You may find some people can't get excited for you right away. People who care about you wonder how this pregnancy will change your life. Others are caught up in their own negative opinions. They worry most about what people will think of you and what people will think of them for being close to you.

There's a good chance at least one person in your life will respond negatively to your pregnancy. For this reason, you need to learn to handle these reactions. There are several things you can do to deal with these responses.

First, accept that not everyone will agree with you. This is hard to do, but it's essential. You will never be able to make everyone happy. You have to make your own decisions based on what you think is best for your life. Just as you have your opinions about what's right, so do others. Disagreeing doesn't make either person right or wrong. It just means you see the situation differently. When someone argues with you, make it clear you accept the person's feelings. You might say, "It's okay for you to disagree with me, but I expect you to respect my decision."

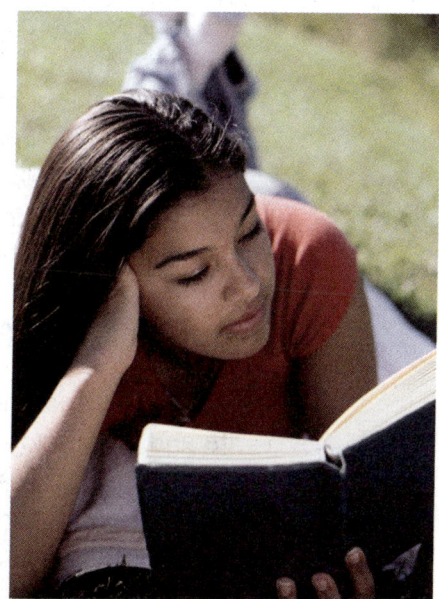

Second, don't take people's negative reactions personally. When people are upset, they often say things they don't mean. They might make hurtful comments or crude remarks. This is most true of first reactions. Don't take these things to heart, especially when they're not true. Feel good about the person you are and the decisions you're making. Don't let anyone make you feel badly about yourself. Find a way to get rid of any bad feelings about what the other person said. Do what works for you, whether it's exercise, writing, or something else you enjoy. See Figure 1-8.

1-8 Taking time to relax can help you deal with the negative reactions of others.

Third, treat the other person with respect no matter how he or she treats you. This may not be easy, but at least you'll have the satisfaction of knowing you have done what's right. Respond in a way that shows your maturity and concern for the other person. If you lower yourself to making rude and hurtful comments, you'll keep the argument going. By refusing to join in, the person may stop sooner. It's okay to stand up for yourself in a firm, but polite way. For instance, you can say, "Don't say those hurtful things to me. That's not helping me."

Preparing to Make a Decision

Admit to yourself that a big decision lies ahead. What will you do regarding your pregnancy? You don't have to decide right now, but it's a good idea to start thinking about it. This pregnancy will not simply go away. At some point, you will need to choose the path you will take. Keeping this in mind can help you prepare for the choice you'll be making. It is also a healthy way to approach the situation.

The Skills You Will Need to Succeed

This series focuses on some of the key skills you'll need as a teen facing pregnancy. You already have some of these skills; you can work to develop the others. The key skills include those needed to make important decisions, build relationships, meet your child's needs, and cope in the outside world. The descriptions given here are an overview. Each skill is discussed more at length in later chapters and books in this series.

Making Decisions

You will soon have to make some important decisions about your life and pregnancy. You can choose to parent, plan an adoption, or have an abortion. You may also need to decide how you can stay in school or keep working. If you parent, you will face decisions about your child's care. You must also choose whether you will marry or parent alone.

The decisions you make will affect your future. Suppose you choose to quit school to stay home with your child. This choice could impact your earning power for the rest of your life. It will be harder to find a decent-paying job without a high school diploma. Your finances will affect you, your child, and any other children you might have in the future.

To make the best decisions, you will need to examine your values, goals, and resources. This skill will help you find out what matters to you, what you want out of life, and what options you have.

Finally, you will need to learn to make wise choices. You'll find the decision-making process helpful. This process involves a few steps you can take to arrive at a decision. Using this process will keep you from making a hasty or uninformed choice. When you make a decision carefully, you will be less likely to regret this choice in the future. This is important. Many of the choices related to pregnancy are permanent. You'll learn more about the decision-making process in Chapter 3.

Building Relationships

Relationships are part of everyday life. You have relationships with many people in your life. This includes your family, friends, neighbors, and classmates. You have a relationship with your child's other parent. How healthy is each of these relationships? Would you like some, or perhaps all, of them to be better? Many skills will help you build relationships.

Increasing your self-esteem is an important relationship skill. Your self-esteem describes the amount of confidence and satisfaction you have in yourself as a person. Do you have a high amount of self-esteem or very little? Your feelings about yourself affect how you relate to others. If you lack self-esteem, it's hard for others to like you. It may be hard for you to make friends if you don't like yourself. You might choose relationships that aren't good for you. On the other hand, when you feel good about yourself, you're more likely to expect the best from relationships. You won't allow others to mistreat you. Your confidence will attract others to you. This makes it easier to make friends.

You will also need communication skills as you relate to others. With these skills, you can understand others and help them to understand you. Many times, you will communicate with words. You can also communicate with the use of messages that don't require words. This might include posture, body language, gestures, tone of voice, and facial expressions. When you communicate, you can learn what the other person feels or thinks. This allows you to get to know this person well. You can also share what you think and how you feel. Good communication skills will help you relate to others in a stronger way.

Be selective about the relationships you enter, too. You couldn't pick your family, but you can choose your friends and dating partners. These are big decisions. You want to choose relationships that will improve your life. See Figure 1-9. Avoid those that will complicate it.

Another relationship skill you will need is being able to deal with conflict. Even in healthy relationships, problems will occur. These conflicts need to be handled. How do you deal with problems?

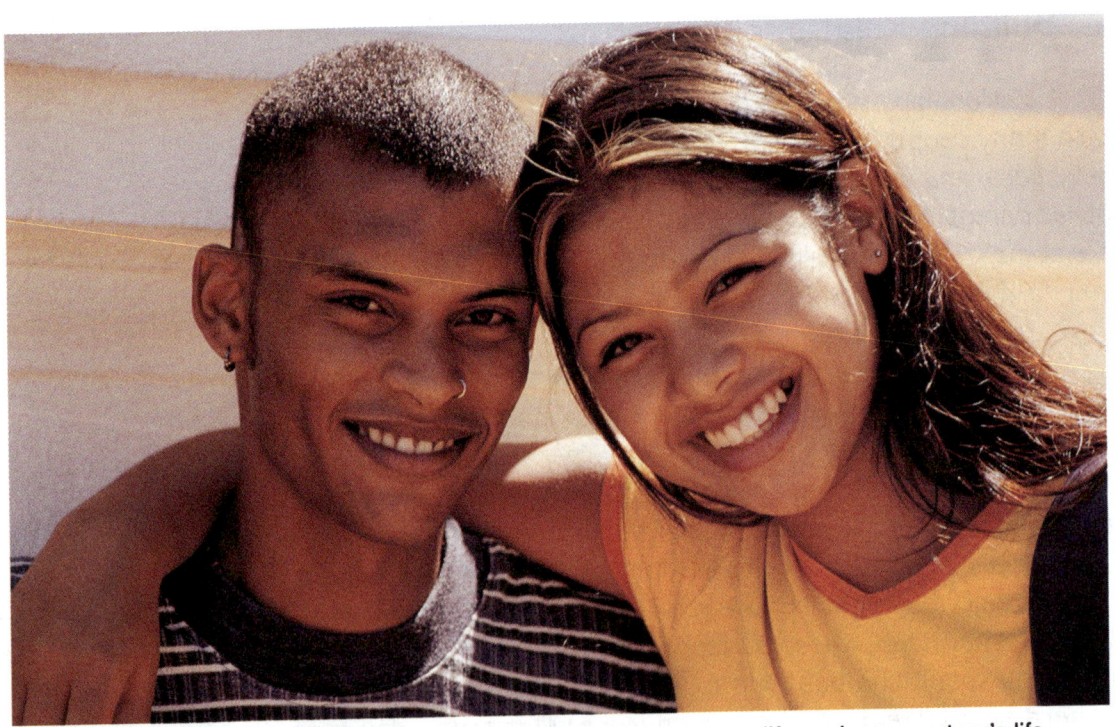

1-9 Choose a healthy dating relationship that will improve your life and your partner's life.

You can flee, fight, or resolve. To *flee* means to run away from the conflict. To *fight* means to try to win the conflict, either verbally or physically. To *resolve* a conflict means to work with the other person to settle the conflict in a way that satisfies you both. Which style of dealing with conflict do you think is the best?

A healthy relationship is one that improves the lives of both people. Sometimes a relationship may start to become less healthy. It may cause you more problems than pleasure. Noticing when this has occurred is a valuable skill. Both of you can choose to make the needed changes in the relationship. What if the other person doesn't want to change? You can choose to end the relationship. This can be difficult. In the long run, though, it's often better than staying in an unhealthy relationship. (More information is given on healthy and unhealthy relationships in later chapters of this book.)

Meeting Your Child's Needs

If you continue your pregnancy, you have a child to consider. Like all children, your child will have many needs in each area of his development. See Figure 1-10. As a parent, it would be your job to meet all these needs to the best of your ability.

Suppose you're deciding whether to parent or plan an adoption. You will want to think about your child's needs and how well you could meet them. You need to understand what is asked of parents before you can know if it's something you can do. Your parenting skills play a large role in your ability to meet a child's needs.

Most parents don't start out with all the skills it takes to meet their children's needs. They have much to learn, and they need a lot of practice. Parenting skills develop over time, but it takes dedication and effort.

Learn as much as you can about children's needs. You can take child development and parenting classes. A second option is to check out books on these subjects from your school or public library. (You can also read more about children's needs in another book in this series, <u>Helping Your Child Grow and Develop</u>.)

What Kinds of Needs Will Your Child Have?

Physical Needs	Intellectual Needs	Social Needs	Emotional Needs
refer to your child's needs for food, clothing, shelter, medical care, rest, and exercise. It will be your job to meet his needs in all these areas. Meeting physical needs often takes money. Being able to provide financially for your child is important. You will also need skills in managing money, being a wise consumer, preparing food, and providing daily care for your child.	refer to your child's need to develop thinking skills. Your child will need you to teach her many things and provide an environment in which she can learn. To grow properly, her brain will need to be stimulated. This stimulation must come from you. You will also be responsible for providing toys and books she can use to learn. Meeting your child's intellectual needs will also mean being ready to learn new things yourself.	refer to your child's need to interact with others. Forming relationships will be an important part of his development. He will first need to build a secure relationship with you. Then, he will need plenty of chances to interact with others. He will need to practice sharing, cooperating, and relating to others. Meeting your child's social needs will also mean teaching him which behaviors are acceptable to the family and society.	refer to your child's need to feel loved and supported. She will need you to constantly show your love for her. You would need to say "I love you" regularly. You could also show affection through kind words, playfulness, hugs, and kisses. Meeting your child's emotional needs will also mean teaching her to express her emotions in a healthy way. This is an important part of being able to get along in the world.

1-10 Children have many needs that parents must meet. Learning about these needs can help you decide whether becoming a parent is right for you.

Coping in the Outside World

As a teen, you're probably used to having your parents handle many things for you. Now that you're pregnant, you may start to do more tasks yourself. This will help you become more independent. For instance, you'll learn to work with professionals in the outside world. These may include health care providers, social service workers, insurance agents, and more. You will learn about resources in your community you did not know existed.

You will have to deal with outside agencies no matter how you handle your pregnancy. If you plan to parent, you might need to talk to someone at your local public aid office. You may be trying to find out whether any financial aid is available to you.

You may not have to do these things all on your own. If your parents are supportive, they may help you. They may share their opinions but encourage you to handle things yourself. They may go with you to medical visits or the social services office, but let you do the talking. If their insurance drops you, they might help you look for a new insurance policy or apply for Medicaid.

Suppose your parents are not this supportive. They may still be upset or opposed to the choice you're making. Your parents may refuse to help. In this case, most of the responsibility will fall on you. If so, ask another relative or trusted adult for help. At school, you might find help from a teacher, nurse, or counselor. A health care provider, social worker, or religious leader may be willing to help, too.

What skills will you need to cope with the outside world? You will need many of the same skills you use to build relationships. Communication and conflict management skills are essential. You will also need to know when and how to seek help. For instance, when you're at your health care provider's office, you may be asked to sign a paper you don't understand. In this case, you need to seek help. Don't sign any paper unless you understand it. Ask someone to explain it to you. (You can learn more about coping with the outside world by reading another book in this series, <u>Building Your Future</u>.)

Major Points

☞ When you learn you're involved in a pregnancy, you may feel overwhelmed with emotion. This is normal. Be patient with yourself as you work to sort things out. If you have thoughts of hurting yourself, seek help right away.

☞ Although it's hard, you need to accept your pregnancy and move on with your life. Ignoring the situation won't make it go away. If you deal with this reality, you can choose what's best for you. Many changes lie ahead of you, but you can adjust to them.

☞ Find someone you can talk to about your pregnancy. Don't tell everyone just yet, though. Start with someone who will be supportive. Think carefully about the right time and way to share this news with others. Prepare yourself to handle any negative reactions that occur.

☞ At this point, you don't need to decide what you will do regarding the pregnancy. You do need to admit to yourself that a big decision lies ahead, though. Keeping this in mind can help you prepare to make this choice. It's also a healthy way to approach the situation.

☞ As a pregnant teen, you will need to enhance certain skills. These skills will help you make important decisions, build relationships, meet your child's needs, and cope with the outside world.

Chapter 2
Improving Your Self-Esteem

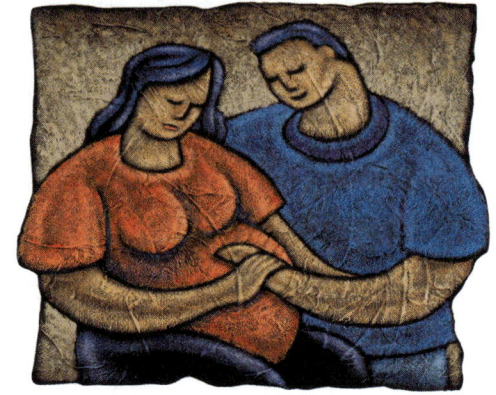

Self-esteem refers to your feelings of confidence and satisfaction with yourself. Some people have a high amount of self-esteem. Others have little or none. In this chapter, you will learn why self-esteem matters. You'll also learn how to evaluate your self-esteem and improve it. This can make your life as a pregnant teen easier. It may help you feel more at ease with the changes you're facing.

What Is Self-Esteem?

Your self-esteem reflects how you <u>feel</u> about yourself and your abilities. This sense of self-esteem develops over time. It is not based on any one day, but is an overall view of yourself.

Your feelings about yourself may fluctuate from day-to-day. You may feel good one day and not as good the next. This is normal. As long as you accept these changes as normal, they shouldn't hurt your self-esteem.

Major life events can affect your self-esteem, though. For instance, you feel a little differently about yourself since you became pregnant. How well you think you're dealing with the pregnancy and the changes it brings will be one factor. Afterward, how you feel about your choices will also play a role. Feeling you handled things poorly can shake your confidence. Handling things well can improve your self-esteem.

Lacking self-esteem means you don't value yourself as a person. You don't feel confident in your skills and abilities. You don't feel able to make a good decision. On the other hand, having self-esteem means you like yourself and have confidence in your skills and abilities. You believe you can make good decisions about your life.

Why Is Self-Esteem Important?

You may wonder why self-esteem matters. Your self-esteem affects many aspects of your life. The effects can be divided into five main groups. These are personal outlook, health and personal care, goals and performance, relationships, and decision making. If you become a parent, your self-esteem will affect your child's life, too.

Personal Outlook

Self-esteem can affect your outlook on life. It can change the way you view yourself and the world. Your self-esteem can help or hurt your chances of living a happy and fulfilled life. It influences your attitude about yourself and your life.

Lacking self-esteem can make it harder for you to find happiness. You may see the world from a negative point of view. For instance, you may overlook the good parts of a situation and see only the bad parts. You see both yourself and others in this way. If you don't like yourself, it's hard for you to like others or have others like you.

Having self-esteem can make it easier for you to find happiness. This means you accept yourself and are pleased with who you are. You'll be more likely to keep a positive attitude. This helps you find the joy in life. Even in bad times, you can see something positive. Focusing on the good side of things helps you maintain your confidence. See Figure 2-1.

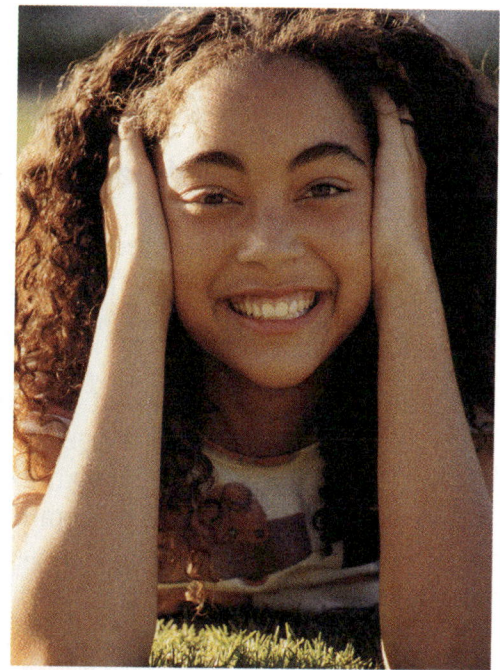

2-1 Having self-esteem makes it easier for you to find happiness by allowing you to focus on the positives in life.

Health and Personal Care

How well you take care of yourself always matters. During pregnancy, though, your health is even more vital. In pregnancy, your health habits will affect not only you, but also the health of your unborn child. Before birth, your baby relies on you to meet all his nutritional needs. Your self-esteem may influence the way you take care of yourself and maintain your health.

Lacking self-esteem means you don't value yourself. This makes it harder to take care of yourself. You may have poor health habits. When your health suffers, it's hard to stay in good spirits. Poor health may reinforce a poor self-image. You may become depressed or feel even worse about yourself than before. In pregnancy, neglecting your health means you and your child will suffer.

Having self-esteem means your health matters to you. You see the value of developing habits that promote good health. You take care of yourself—getting the exercise, nutrition, and rest you need. Good health can help you keep a positive outlook, which can strengthen self-esteem. In pregnancy, your child has the best chance for a healthy start when you meet your own health needs.

Goals and Performance

Self-esteem can affect your ability to set and meet goals. It also plays a role in performance at school and on the job. Your self-esteem can influence your ability to handle rough tasks and adjust to changes.

Lacking self-esteem means you don't think enough of yourself to form a plan for success. You may not understand why goals are important. Without self-esteem, you may not think you can achieve. This can make it hard to set realistic goals. Instead, you may set goals that are too easy or too hard to achieve. Goals that are too easy don't challenge you to reach your potential. Goals that are too hard may be impossible to achieve, which might reinforce your lack of self-esteem.

Lacking self-esteem can also affect your performance in school and on the job. If you don't like yourself, it's hard to be enthused about anything you're doing. You may have a "who cares" attitude.

At school, this attitude can lead to poor grades, which will only reinforce your lack of self-esteem. If you don't believe in yourself, you're less likely to put forth the effort it takes to succeed. You may not be able to handle rough tasks or adjust to changes well.

When you have self-esteem, you know why goals are important. You can see them as steps on the way to achieving your plans and dreams. You're able to set goals that are realistic. These goals are challenging but possible to achieve. When you believe in yourself, you're willing to put in the effort it takes to succeed in school. See Figure 2-2. You feel confident the hard work will pay off. You see rough tasks as obstacles that can be overcome, and change as a normal part of life.

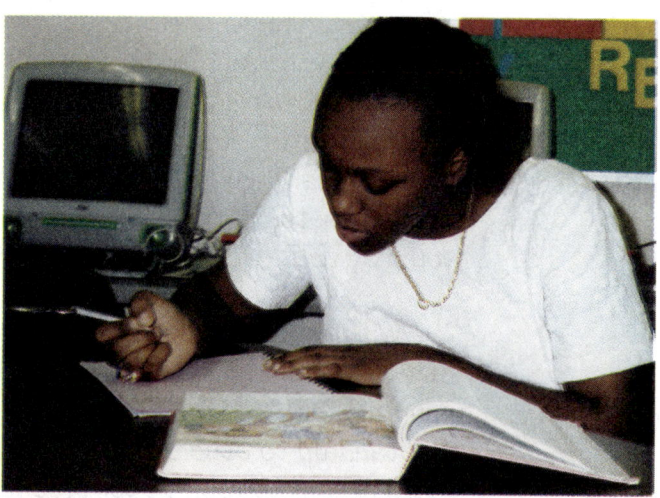

2-2 When you have self-esteem, you will work hard to succeed in everything you do. You realize finishing school is an important goal to achieve.

Decision Making

The amount of self-esteem you have can affect your ability to make good decisions. If you lack self-esteem, you may be more likely to make poor decisions. You may not have confidence in your decision making. You may think things in your life always turn out for the worst. If so, you might be afraid to put a lot of time and effort into decision making. When you don't care much about yourself, you might make a hasty decision. You are more likely to regret this kind of decision in the future.

When you have self-esteem, you want the best for yourself. You can see how important it is to make the best choice. You value yourself enough to take the time to carefully think things through. As a pregnant teen, you will face many big decisions. If you believe in yourself, you'll be more likely to make wise decisions and be satisfied with them. You'll have fewer regrets later in life.

Relationships

Your self-esteem will affect your relationships with others. It may determine the types of friends you have. How you allow people to treat you also tells a lot about your self-esteem.

When you don't value yourself, it shows. Others may pick up on your lack of self-esteem. Also, people with little self-esteem often have a negative outlook. These people are unhappy much of the time. It can be hard to have fun with someone who's always down. If you lack self-esteem, this can make it harder to find friends. As a result, you may settle for unhealthy relationships.

Without self-esteem, you're also more likely to be mistreated by others. Accepting abuse sends the message you don't think much of yourself. Perhaps you don't think you deserve more. You may be scared to stand up to others for fear of losing key relationships. This can make it hard to resist peer pressure. Following others can sometimes have negative results.

When you have self-esteem, it may be easier to make friends. Your confidence, positive outlook, and sense of happiness will draw others to you. These qualities will make you more pleasant to be around.

Having self-esteem also means you want only the best for yourself. You see the value of choosing relationships wisely. People who have self-esteem don't settle for being mistreated. Instead they expect others to treat them well. This shows they respect themselves and care about what happens to them. If you have self-esteem, it will be easier for you to have healthy relationships with others.

Parenting

Self-esteem matters when it comes to parenting, too. If you decide to parent, your self-esteem will affect your child. To feel effective as a parent, you have to first believe in yourself. You need to trust yourself to decide what's right for your child. This requires self-esteem.

Your self-esteem may influence how you will treat your child. When you love and respect yourself, it's easier to love and respect someone else. Improving your self-esteem can help you become a more loving parent. This can make your child feel more valued and boost her self-esteem.

You will be your child's first and most important role model. She'll learn much by watching you. Your attitude will set an example she'll be likely to follow. If you see yourself and the world in a negative light, so will she. Your child may pick up on your lack of hope and confidence. She may feel this way about herself, too. Having self-esteem helps you see the best in yourself and the world. Showing your child you care about yourself will set a positive example. It may give her a good start on forming her own self-esteem.

Having self-esteem means wanting only the best for yourself. This includes choosing healthy habits and relationships. When you do this, your child receives the added benefit of a healthy home environment. Here she can feel nurtured and supported. This will help her develop her own sense of self-esteem. In this way, improving your self-esteem boosts your child's self-esteem, too.

How Is Self-Esteem Formed?

Believe it or not, your self-esteem has been shaped from the moment you were born. See Figure 2-3. How a parent held you, spoke to you, and cared for you gave the first messages you had about yourself. If those messages were positive, they may have helped you feel good about yourself. This built your self-esteem. Suppose the messages were negative. This could have damaged your self-esteem.

You may have felt your parents' love and respect for you. If so, this may have helped you learn to value yourself. If you felt unloved or unwanted by your parents, it might have lead you to feel less satisfied with who you are.

Parents aren't the only family members who affect your self-esteem. Brothers and sisters also play a role. They might have always picked on you or put you down. This could have hurt your self-esteem. On the other hand, if they loved and supported you, it would boost your self-esteem. Aunts, uncles, cousins, and grandparents affect your self-esteem, too. If these family members praise and compliment you, it can help you feel good about yourself.

In a healthy family, each member tries to help and support the others. This isn't true of all families, though. When families don't love and support each other, it may damage the members' sense of worth.

Experiences can also shape your self-esteem. How well you've gotten along with others at school and in the community is one factor. If you've been able to make friends easily, this boosts your

How Was Your Self-Esteem Formed?

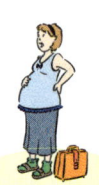

Pregnancy. Teen pregnancy can change the way you see yourself. How you're handling things matters, too.

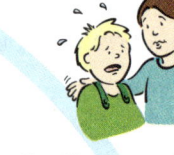

Parents. How your parents treated you helped shape your self-esteem.

Major life events. Important events, such as moving to a new place or losing a family member to death, can affect your self-esteem.

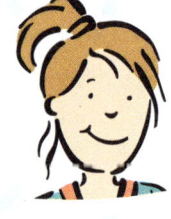

Brothers and sisters. If your siblings were supportive, this may have raised your self-esteem.

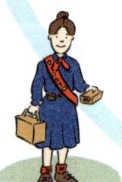

Community. Getting along with others and participating in community events and organizations can affect your self-esteem.

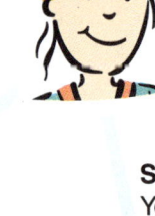

School. Your experiences and performance in school can strengthen or harm your self-esteem.

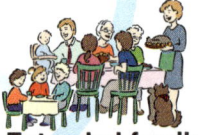

Extended family. Your cousins, aunts, uncles, and grandparents have influenced the way you see yourself.

 This diagram shows several influences on self-esteem. How have these influenced your self-esteem?

self-esteem. If you feel left out by others, this may have lowered your opinion of yourself. How your friends treat you also affects your self-esteem.

Your performance in school can help or harm your self-esteem. Finding talents and being able to use them makes you feel good. Struggling with schoolwork can shake your confidence. Teachers may have boosted your self-esteem or damaged it.

Experiences in activities outside school also play a role. In these activities, how you were treated by others and how well you've performed can affect your view of yourself. If you went out for sports and played well, this could help. Suppose you went out for sports and sat on the bench the entire season. This may have affected your feelings about yourself in a less positive way.

If key adults in these activities supported you, this could boost your self-esteem. A youth group leader who took the time to listen would make you feel important. If a recreation leader chose you as team captain, this would show confidence in your ability to lead others. These responses would have raised your self-esteem. Less positive interactions might have damaged it.

When you were a young child, your basic sense of self-esteem was shaped. Your experiences, however, can gradually change your self-esteem. Events in your life may affect how you feel about yourself. This can be a positive or negative influence. Major life events that might affect your self-esteem include the following:

- ☛ changing schools
- ☛ moving to a new neighborhood
- ☛ having a divorce or death in your family

Pregnancy is an event that may affect your self-esteem. How you feel about being pregnant can change your view of yourself. You may feel pregnancy brings a greater importance to your life. Instead, you may feel you have made a big mistake and ruined your life. You can see how each of these reactions could affect your self-esteem.

In pregnancy, you face rough tasks and must adjust to many changes. If you feel good about how you're handling things, it can boost your self-esteem. See Figure 2-4. If not, this might lower your confidence.

Evaluating Your Self-Esteem

Now you know what self-esteem is, why it matters, and how it is formed. You may wonder how you can use this information. Understanding these concepts can help you measure your own self-esteem. Evaluating your self-esteem can help you know yourself better. You will have a clearer idea of who you are and how you feel about yourself. This can help you make changes for the better.

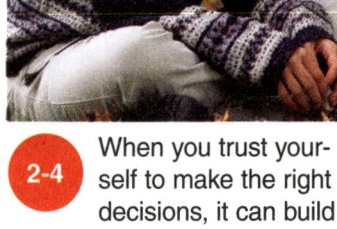

2-4 When you trust yourself to make the right decisions, it can build your self-esteem.

It can be hard to judge your own self-esteem. When you feel good, you may think you have a high amount of self-esteem. On a bad day, you might think your self-esteem has slipped to a low level. In reality, these feelings may only be a passing mood swing. Your true self-esteem changes very gradually.

Choose a time when you're feeling about average to examine your self-esteem. You can start by taking several minutes to relax and think. What kind of feelings do you have about yourself? What sorts of images come to mind? This will get you started.

You might want to create some lists involving self-esteem. For instance, list all the good points you can identify about yourself. Do the same for negative qualities. Which list is longer? This may give you some idea how satisfied you are with yourself as a person. Draw a line across the length of a sheet of paper. Label one end <u>high amount of self-esteem</u> and the other end <u>low amount of self-esteem</u>. Where on this scale do you think you fall? From time to time, draw a circle showing your position on this line. This may tell you if your sense of self-esteem is changing.

Another way to explore your self-esteem is to talk to a trusted friend who knows you very well. Ask this person his or her opinion regarding your self-esteem. Does your friend think you possess self-esteem or lack it? What makes him or her form this conclusion? Are there signs you show? These signs may be obvious to someone else, but difficult for you to notice. In discussing your self-esteem with this friend, what have you learned about yourself?

You can also evaluate your self-esteem by using a self-assessment tool. This is a list of questions somewhat like a quiz. The questions focus on how you feel about yourself. Honest answers can reveal your level of self-esteem. This type of quiz can also point out the areas where you can make positive changes. You might like to use an informal assessment like the one shown in Figure 2-5. You can also ask your counselor or teacher to help you find a more formal self-assessment. He or she can help you interpret your results. This person might be able to help you work through your feelings about the results.

How Can You Improve Your Self-Esteem?

You will probably discover that, even if you have self-esteem, you can still improve it. What this means is you have room to grow. If you want to build your self-esteem, there are many ways you can do so.

Get to Know Yourself

The best way to enhance your self-esteem is to learn more about yourself. Spend more time thinking about what you want and need. Find ways to meet these wants and needs. Take the time to do things you enjoy. See Figure 2-6. Focus on working to become a better and stronger person. Your efforts will pay off. As you become more satisfied, you will see yourself in a better light. This will boost your self-esteem.

Use Positive Self-Talk

You can also improve your self-esteem through positive self-talk. The messages you send yourself about you are called self-talk. Everyone uses self-talk. Positive self-talk focuses on your strengths and successes. When self-talk is negative, it describes faults and failures. Negative self-talk can damage your self-esteem. Learn to talk to yourself in positive ways.

Examining Your Self-Esteem

As you read each statement, place a check in the column to the right that describes how often the statement is true of you. (There are no right or wrong answers.) For now, leave the Score column blank.

	Always	Usually	Sometimes	Never	Score
1. Do you feel good about yourself?					
2. Are you confident in your ability to succeed?					
3. Do you feel confident in your ability to make the best decision?					
4. Do you carefully think things through before making an important decision?					
5. Are you satisfied with who you are?					
6. Do you respect yourself as a person?					
7. Do you accept your weaknesses and flaws?					
8. Can you own up to your mistakes and learn from them?					
9. Do you make friends easily?					
10. Do you have a positive attitude most of the time?					
11. Do you focus on the good parts of a bad situation?					
12. Are you happy, or at least content, most of the time?					
13. Do you do the best work you can at school and/or work?					
14. Do you set realistic goals for yourself?					
15. Do you get enough food, sleep, and exercise?					
16. Do you try to keep yourself healthy?					
17. Do you choose relationships that are healthy for you?					
18. Do you expect others to treat you well?					
19. Are you able to stand up for yourself when problems occur in a relationship?					
20. Would you end a relationship that is no longer healthy if the other person refused to change his or her behavior?					
Use this key to rate each of your answers: Always = 3 points; Usually = 2 points; Sometimes = 1 point; and Never = 0 points. Record your answer for each question in the Score column on the far right side of the page. When you have scored all responses, add the scores. Record the answer in the Total box. Sixty points are possible.				Total	

2-5 Use this checklist as an informal assessment of your self-esteem. Does your score surprise you?

You can also use self-talk when someone says something negative to you. For example, if someone says you're not a good parent, you may be hurt or angry. You might think the person is right. (This is an example of negative self-talk.) Instead, tell yourself, "I know I'm not perfect, but I'm working hard to be the best parent I can be." This is positive self-talk. Reminding yourself of your good points can enhance your self-esteem.

Learning to use positive self-talk is not always easy. You may not even be aware of all the negative self-talk you use. It may be more of a habit than you think. For a few days, focus on all the times you use negative self-talk. Keep track on a sheet of paper. Was this problem bigger or smaller than you had thought?

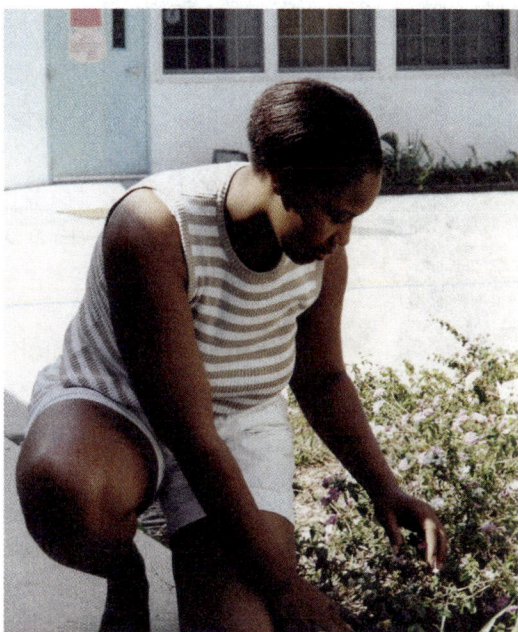

2-6 Spending more time doing things you enjoy, such as gardening, can help you get to know yourself better. This can raise your self-esteem.

Starting to use positive self-talk may mean changing some behaviors you have used all your life. It will take time, practice, and patience. Set a goal to replace negative self-talk with positive self-talk. This goal should be realistic and measurable. For instance, your first goal might be to listen for negative self-talk and follow each negative message with three positive ones.

Write your goal on paper and read it several times a day. Keep the paper in a place you will see it often. This will keep your goal fresh in your mind. Record notes about how well you're meeting your goal. Once you feel confident with this goal, set another, bigger one. In this way, you can work to slowly rid your life of negative self-talk and replace it with positive self-talk. This will improve your self-esteem.

Learn to Visualize Success

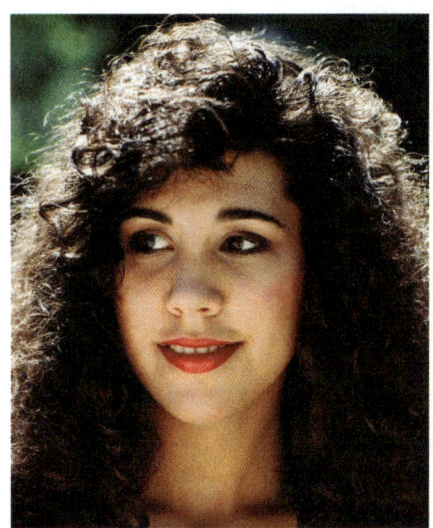

2-7 Visualize what it would be like if you had already accomplished your goal. Use this image to encourage you.

To visualize means to form an image in your mind. When you visualize success, you picture yourself reaching your goals. You imagine doing whatever it is you want to do. See Figure 2-7. If you visualize school success, you might see your test marked with a good grade. You can use this as a tool to raise your self-esteem.

Try using this technique. Choose an area in which you want to improve. Set a goal stating how you will do this. Now, visualize yourself reaching this goal. Close your eyes and pretend you can see yourself succeeding. Walk yourself through the goal step-by-step. By visualizing success, you can help yourself believe it is possible. This can give you the confidence you need to achieve your goal. In turn, meeting goals will further boost your confidence and enhance your self-esteem.

Talk with a Professional

A professional can also help you work to develop your self-esteem. You might want to see a social worker or counselor. These people have been trained to help people work through their problems. They can guide you as you learn more about yourself and work to build self-esteem.

Gaining self-esteem through counseling is not a quick process. It happens over time. As you form a relationship with your counselor, he or she learns more about you. Then he or she can offer suggestions that will fit your needs.

You can find counselors and social workers in most communities. Some may offer counseling for little or no cost. Your teacher or school counselor may be able to help you find someone who works with teens.

In some small communities, a counselor or social worker may not be available. Also, some people have religious beliefs that do not allow them to go to counseling. Others can't afford to see a counselor. If you are in one of these situations, talk with a trusted adult. This might be a religious leader, teacher, or a caseworker from the public aid office. This person may be able to assist you with problems. Talking about your feelings can help. A trusted adult can help you see the good in yourself. This will build your self-esteem.

Strengthen Your Support System

To boost your self-esteem, you can strengthen your support system. Your support system is the network of people and organizations you can rely on in times of need. This support system includes your family members, friends, and other important people in your life. It can include school and medical personnel. A professional counselor can also be a support for you. If you feel supported and loved, your self-esteem will increase. You'll see others think you're valuable and remind yourself that you should, too.

Surround yourself with people who will lift your spirits rather than bring you down. See Figure 2-8. Find people you can talk to about your feelings and what's going on in your life. If you need to develop some new friendships, take the time and energy to do this. It will help you feel supported.

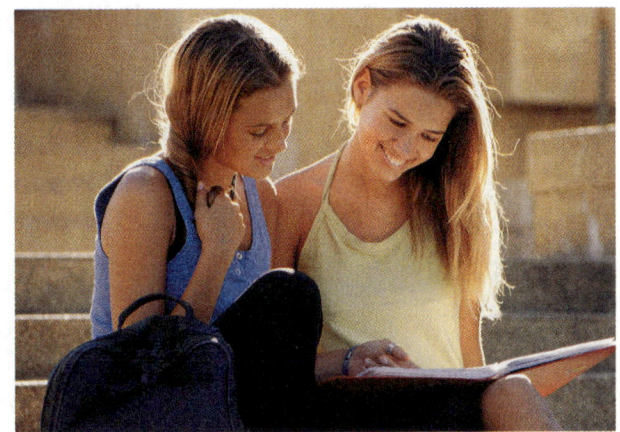

2-8 Having a strong support system that includes good friends will make you feel better about yourself.

One way to strengthen your support system is to join a support group. This is a group of people who share a similar challenge or concern. In a support group, members talk about their concerns. They offer support to one another. Many support groups have an adult leader, who is called a facilitator. Some support groups are led by teens. Support groups are usually free of charge.

Your school or community may have a support group for pregnant and parenting teens. Most communities have many others as well. Talk to your school counselor about support groups available in your area. If no support group is offered for pregnant and parenting teens, think about starting one. You may want to find an adult volunteer to lead the group.

Support groups help you build self-esteem by creating a safe environment for you. They help you feel comfortable talking about the challenges you face. This can help you realize you're not alone—others have felt your same concerns. When you feel supported in this way, you may value yourself more. You might be less likely to blame yourself for what has happened to you.

You can learn from the others in your support group. They can share what has worked for them when they faced a situation like yours. This can teach you new ways to address your concerns. In a support group, you can also talk to other members about the problems you've faced in the past. Helping others can make you feel good, which can raise your self-esteem.

Take Responsibility for Your Life

Taking responsibility for your life can also increase your self-esteem. This will give you a sense of power regarding your life. You'll learn you can make decisions about what's best for you and carry them out. This can make you feel good about yourself.

When you take responsibility, it means you play an active role in your life. You make the decisions and do what needs to be done to see them through. This means you own all your successes and failures. You understand that people make mistakes, and you accept yourself for who you are. This is much healthier than running away from your problems or blaming others.

When you blame others, you don't accept the role you played in the problem. You focus on the other person's mistakes and talk about him or her in a negative way. It can make you feel badly to blame someone else for something you know was really your fault. Not admitting your mistakes means you can't learn and grow from them. If you don't learn from mistakes, you are likely to repeat them.

Blaming others is much easier than admitting fault. Taking responsibility is the more mature approach. This means claiming your mistakes and learning from them. In this way, you can grow as a person and learn to celebrate your successes. Taking responsibility for yourself will improve your self-esteem.

Major Points

- Self-esteem refers to your feelings of confidence and satisfaction with yourself. It reflects your feelings about yourself and your abilities.

- Self-esteem is important for a number of reasons. It affects your personal outlook, health and personal care habits, goals and performance, decision making, and relationships. If you lack self-esteem, it can lead to problems in each of these areas. Having self-esteem is linked to better outcomes in each area.

- If you parent, self-esteem will influence your parenting skills and how you treat your child. Having self-esteem sets a good example and improves your relationship with your child. Lacking self-esteem can affect your child's self-esteem and the way you treat her.

- Self-esteem develops gradually in a process that begins at birth. It is influenced by your relationships with important people in your life, especially your family. As you grow, experiences can also affect your self-esteem.

- Evaluating your self-esteem can give you an idea of where you stand. It can help you know yourself better and make plans for improvement. You can evaluate your self-esteem in informal or formal ways.

- Increasing your self-esteem can improve your life. You can gain self-esteem in many ways. Some ideas are getting to know yourself, using positive self-talk, learning to visualize success, talking with a professional, strengthening your support system, and taking responsibility for your life.

Chapter 3
Considering Values, Goals, and Decisions

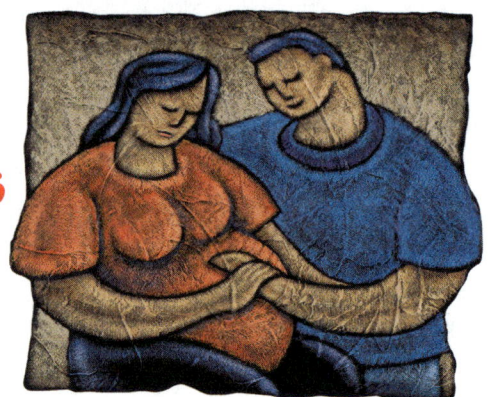

Many important decisions lie ahead for you. At first, these decisions may seem overwhelming. Have confidence in yourself—you can do it! This chapter will give you some of the guidance you need. You will learn about the decision-making process. This is a step-by-step method of making decisions. This chapter will also teach you about values and goals. You will need to consider these when making a decision. With these tools, you can make the decisions that are best for you.

Values

Your values are your beliefs, feelings, and ideas about what is important. Values can't be seen or touched, but they influence how you live. Your values will guide your behavior as you work to meet your needs. Values are the foundation of your goals and decisions. This means you will set goals and make decisions based on what you think is important.

You may have many different types of values. For instance, honesty, openness, and happiness are examples of values. You might also value education, religious beliefs, and financial security. Time spent with your friends and family might be important to you, too. Your values tell what matters most to you. Figure 3-1 lists more values you might have.

Many of your actions are based on your personal values. If you value education, it would bother you to skip school. You would consider this value if friends asked you to skip school with them. If

Chapter 3   Considering Values, Goals, and Decisions

school is important to you, you might try to go to school even when you don't feel well. You might think about how much your grades or learning matters to you.

Even when you don't think about values, they can guide your actions. Over time, it may become more natural for your actions to reflect your values. Suppose you value honesty. You may not even think about whether to answer test questions without cheating. In this case, honesty may just be automatic for you.

How Are Values Developed?

Your original set of values probably came from your family. Your parents have been teaching you what matters most to them. Other factors will shape your values, too. Some of these are friends, the media, religious beliefs, and school. Your experiences and choices can also have an effect.

What Do You Value?

- teamwork
- knowledge
- independence
- creativity
- patriotism
- family unity
- prestige
- fitness
- power
- health
- self-discipline
- friendship
- dating/marriage relationship
- money
- financial security
- job (career)
- hard work
- education
- honesty
- fairness
- openness
- love
- respect
- equality
- patience
- religious beliefs
- sports
- appearance
- fashion
- material objects (such as car, stereo, computer)
- competition
- responsibility
- taking care of others
- loyalty

3-1 Which of these values are important to you? What others do you hold?

Family Influences

As a young child, you began learning about values from your parents. All your life, they've been teaching you about the values they hold. Some of these lessons are direct, while others are indirect. For instance, when your parents told you it was good to share with others, this was a direct lesson. You could have also learned about the value of sharing indirectly, by watching your parents share with others.

How your parents responded to your behavior taught you about their values. When you were a child, if your parents rewarded a behavior, you learned they valued it. If they punished or ignored a behavior, you saw this behavior wasn't valued. When parents are consistent, children can learn their parents' values. Although your values may change somewhat over time, most people adopt the values of their families, at least initially.

Influences of Friends

Friends also influence your values. Most children and teens want to be like their friends because they want to fit in. At school, if a child watches the teacher praise a friend for sharing toys, it will influence him to share. Both the teacher and the other child have influenced him. Teens often want to dress like their friends. They value friendship and believe how they dress will influence who their friends will be.

You will also spend a lot of time with your friends. See Figure 3-2. As a result, you'll be exposed to their values. You might adopt some of these values as an attempt to belong. This could have either a positive or negative effect. If your

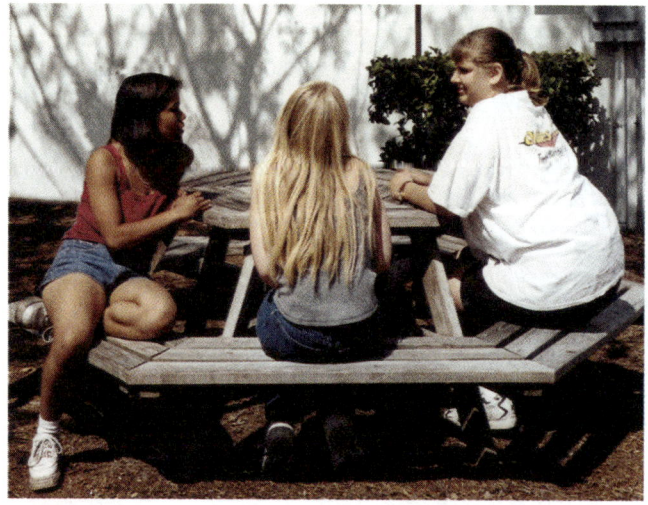

3-2 Friends can influence your values. As you spend time talking with friends, you learn more about what their values are.

friends have values that promote your well-being, these could be a good influence. Some of their values might hurt you. For instance, you might have friends who value thrill-seeking behaviors. If you spend lots of time with these friends, you might be injured or get into trouble.

Media Influences

Today, the media has a big influence on values. Some forms of the media are TV, movies, music, and magazines. You may have seen TV programs and movies that were not realistic. Often, the values they show are not ones that society accepts. You may see people who lie, cheat, and steal. They may act in violent ways or use drugs. If you watch these programs or movies, you might think these values are accepted. You might even adopt some of them. The same can be true of some of the music you hear and music videos you see.

Magazines may shape your values by the models they feature. A fashion magazine might show the values of beauty, youth, and fitness. These magazines value being very thin and wearing the latest fashions, too. If you adopt these values, you might be disappointed, though. Not many people can afford to buy all the most popular styles of clothing. Very few women are as thin as the models in the magazines. Trying to be this thin can cause health problems. It can lead to an addiction to excessive exercise, an unhealthy body image, or an eating disorder. This can be dangerous.

Religious Influences

The religious beliefs you have may also help shape your values. Each religious group has its own set of beliefs. If you belong to a house of worship, you'll learn the values of that group. You may adopt some of these values as your own. For instance, many religious groups encourage people to treat others as they would like to be treated. Treating others well is a value you might learn and adopt through your religious group.

School Influences

The schools you attend may shape your values. Both the students and teachers at school set examples you can learn to follow. See Figure 3-3. School personnel also respond to your behavior in a way that teaches you right from wrong behavior. This can also influence your values. Finally, the knowledge you gain at school may help you see life differently. Some of your values may come from what you have learned in school.

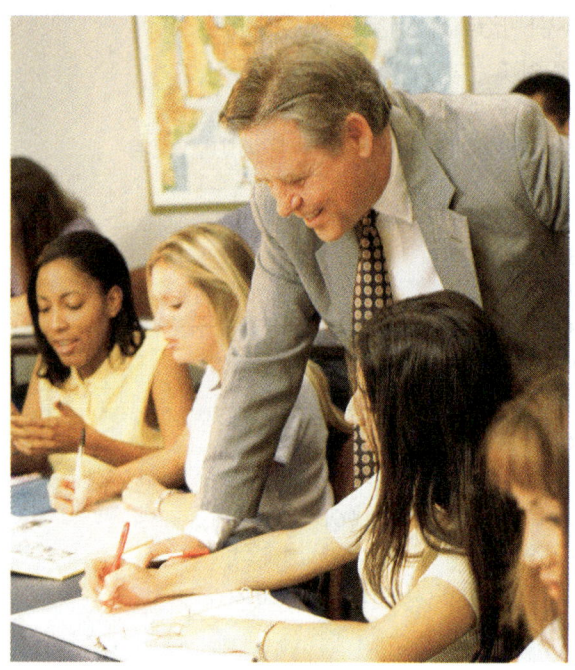

3-3 Teachers can set an example for their students of the importance of helping others. This can influence a student's values.

Personal Experiences and Choices

Experiences can also change your values. For instance, pregnancy may cause you to change some of your values. Before you were pregnant, you may have valued after-school activities and time with friends. During your pregnancy, health and decision making are more important. If you decide to parent your child, your values will likely change even more. Parenting comes first, but education is important, too. After-school activities and time with friends may have to take a backseat. You may not have to give them up totally—but your time and energy must go to parenting and education first.

All these factors may influence your values. However, it's up to you to decide whether you'll accept or reject these influences. Ultimately, you're the one who determines what your values will be. You will reap the rewards or suffer the consequences of the values you hold. Monitoring your actions and values may make you more aware of changes you might want to make in your values.

Chapter 3   Considering Values, Goals, and Decisions   55

Value Conflicts

A *value conflict* describes tension that occurs when two values or sets of values are in disagreement. You may have a value conflict with someone whose values differ from yours. It's also possible to have a value conflict within yourself. This happens if you hold two competing values. You might also be influenced to adopt values that differ from yours.

Conflicts may occur when two or more people have different values. For example, parents sometimes disagree over how to discipline their children. They may not share the same values and beliefs about raising children. For instance, consider that many young children fight with one another sometimes until they learn better ways to settle problems. Suppose one parent thinks a child should fight back if hit by another child. The other parent might believe hitting others is never okay. This is a value conflict, and it can give the child mixed messages. One parent values pride and defending oneself. The other values peace and nonviolence. Their child may feel confused and unsure about how to act in this situation.

Resolving this type of conflict can be a challenge. No matter what the conflict is, both people should talk about their values on the subject. Respect each other's values and ideas even if you don't agree. Next, decide what matters most to both of you about the outcome of this situation. Knowing this will help you set a common goal. Each of you may need to compromise to reach the goal. This means working to find a solution that satisfies everyone. To meet this common goal, both of you may have to give up some of what you wanted. However, despite the value conflict, you will have worked together to solve the most important part of the problem.

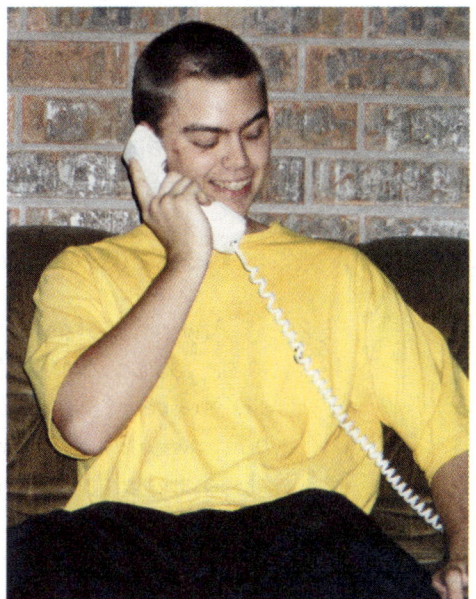

3-4   Value conflicts may occur when your values, such as spending time talking on the phone with friends, conflict with those of your parents.

Suppose one of your top values is time spent with friends. You might spend a long time each night on the phone with your friends. See Figure 3-4. What if your parents have family time as one of their top values? This is a value conflict. Perhaps you and your parents could talk about the situation and come to an agreement. You might have to limit your phone use sometimes. Your parents might have to settle for less family time than they would like. This would help your family resolve the value conflict in a way that satisfies everyone.

A value conflict can also happen within a person. For example, you may value both friendship and education. Suppose a friend asks you to skip class to see a movie. You may feel a value conflict. You want to be with your friend, but you also want to graduate from high school.

Value conflicts can occur when you learn one set of values at home and another set at school or in society. If this happens, you may not know which values to follow. This can make it harder for you to succeed. It might lead you to get into trouble.

Suppose you want to solve a value conflict within yourself. You need to prioritize, which means to decide what is most important. If something is a priority, it is of greater importance to you than other things. To prioritize your values, you will rank them in order of importance. The most important one is your top priority. When choosing among competing values, decide which value you feel takes priority. Make the choice that best supports this value.

How Are Values Changed?

Any of the factors that influence you to form a value can also cause you to change it. Your family or friends may play a part. Your religious beliefs and life experiences can affect your values, too. As you grow and learn more about the world, you may adopt some new values and adjust others.

From time to time, you may notice a certain value no longer matters to you as much as it once did. Perhaps another value is now more important than before. Identifying that a change is needed is a good first step. It means you are in touch with yourself and your needs.

The second step is to review your present values and adjust your priorities. In this step, think about what you have valued in life. What has been most important to you? In reflecting on this, you will note where problems are or if change is needed. Then you can adjust your priorities to include the values you now feel should be most important.

Third, you need to bring your actions into line with your values. Some of your old habits and behaviors may not fit your adjusted value system. You will need to change or eliminate these. Replace them with habits and behaviors that support the values you have chosen now. This step will take time and dedication. Effort and practice are also needed to change the way you act.

For instance, you may decide to put a higher value on your education. You may focus on your graduation. With a diploma, you're more likely to find a job that can support you (and your child, if you become a parent). The next step is to set new priorities that put education first. Change any behaviors that don't support your education. Politely say no if your friends ask you to skip class. Think about how this would interfere with your education. Add some new behaviors that <u>do</u> support your values. You might try studying more, reading chapters more carefully, and keeping up with your homework.

Goals and Resources

A goal is a statement of something you want to accomplish. Two types of goals are short-term and long-term goals. A short-term goal is a plan to accomplish something soon, perhaps within a month or two. A long-term goal is a plan to achieve something in a longer period of time, perhaps a year, five years, or more. Planning to earn a degree in computer programming is a long-term goal. See Figure 3-5. Getting a good grade on next week's test would be a short-term goal.

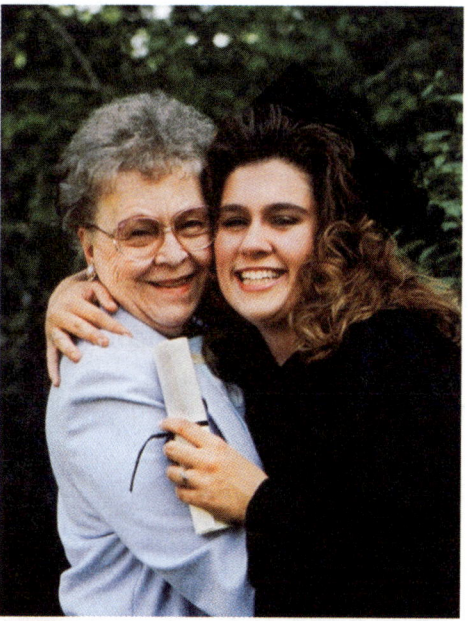

3-5 Graduating from high school is a long-term goal because it takes four years to reach this goal.

Goals are important because they give you a sense of direction. Without goals, you would be much like a driver without a road map. You'd have no clear picture of where you're headed or how you will get there. Goals are plans for turning your hopes and dreams into reality. Setting goals will greatly increase your chances of success.

Goals Are Often Based on Values

The goals you set are based on your values. You might set different goals if your top value is education than if it were sports. Goals that reflect your values are the easiest to reach. These goals will help you accomplish what you feel is important in life. Goals that are unrelated to your values may be harder to achieve. It may be tough to justify your efforts to meet these goals.

You need to set both long- and short-term goals related to your values. This will help you do the work needed to accomplish them. Suppose you value education. Your long-term goal might be to go to college to earn a degree in teaching. You might set three related short-term goals to help you meet this larger goal. These might be to

- attend class every day
- complete your assignments every day
- join a study group

Can you see how your short- and long-term goals can fit together? By reaching the short-term goals, you're taking steps toward your long-term goal. These steps will help you meet that goal.

Resources Help You Reach Goals

Resources are the means you have for reaching your goals. If you manage your resources wisely, they can help you accomplish your goals. There are three main types of resources. Some resources can be touched and seen, while others cannot.

Human resources are those that come from within a person. Each person has human resources that are unique to him or her. Some examples are time, skills, talents, education, wisdom, and energy. Using your time wisely will help you meet your goals. Other personal traits can serve as resources, too. Sometimes you can count other people as human resources, too. Your teachers, parents, and friends may give their time, wisdom, and energy to help you meet your goals.

A second type of resources is **material resources**. These include your money and all the items you possess. Material resources can help you meet goals. For instance, if your goal is to excel in tennis, you will need a racket and some clothing suited for tennis. These are material resources. The money needed to buy these items is also a material resource. Another example is the telephone. You can use the phone to gain information or access other resources. See Figure 3-6. What material resources do you have? Can you see how you could use these to reach your goals?

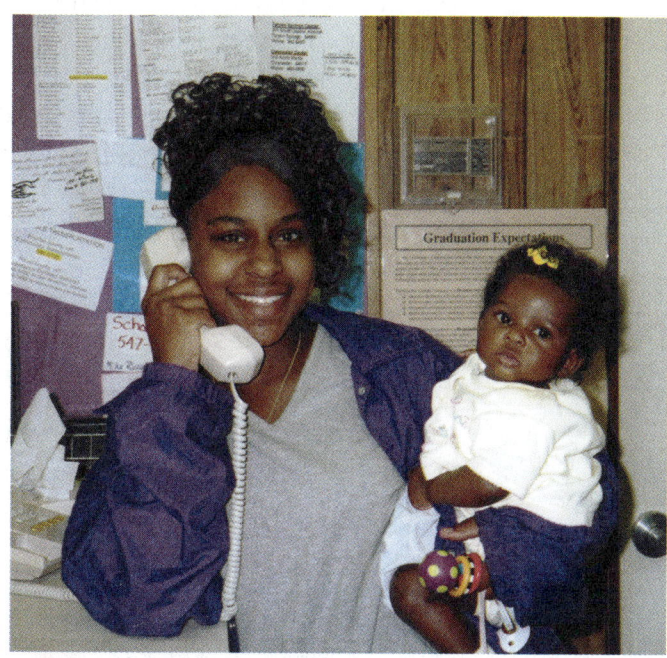

3-6 You can use the telephone to arrange appointments or gather information. This is an example of a material resource

A third type of resources is **community resources**. A person can access these resources just by being part of his or her community. For instance, you have access to public buildings and parks in your town or city. You can use community services, too. These include schools, libraries, health departments, and police departments. Local tax dollars go to support these services for all the members of the community.

How can you use community resources to help you reach your goal? Taking a parenting class offered by your community could help you as a new parent. This might help you meet a goal of learning more parenting skills. If your goal is to write a term paper, you might do research at the public library. To get into shape, you might jog or walk in your city park.

How you manage your resources is important. It has a large effect on your ability to reach your goals. Resources are limited. The resources you use for one purpose cannot be used for another purpose. What if your goal is to save money for college tuition? If you use your money to buy a car, you cannot put these same dollars toward your savings goal. Perhaps your goal is to study two hours each night. To meet this goal, you must devote your human resources (time and energy) to it. If you spend time on the phone with friends, you cannot get these minutes back and use them to study. Putting your resources to their best use will help you reach your goals.

You Can Learn How to Set Goals

The first step in setting a goal is to decide what you want to accomplish. After stating your proposed goal, consider the following questions:

- Is this goal in line with my values? (If not, you may wish to revise the goal to fit better with your values.)
- What will I gain by reaching this goal? How will I feel when I accomplish it?
- Does this goal involve any risks? Is reaching the goal worth taking these risks?
- Is this goal realistic? (Setting a goal that is impossible to reach will only set you up for disappointment. A realistic goal is one that is within your power to achieve.)
- Is this goal specific? (A vague goal is hard to measure. You may not be sure when you've reached it. When setting a specific goal, include a time frame and a way to measure the outcome. This will help you evaluate your progress. See Figure 3-7.)

Now that you've clarified your goal, write it on a sheet of paper. You're ready to proceed with the planning step. What will you need to do to achieve this goal? Can you break the goal into subgoals to help you achieve it? Subgoals are smaller, related steps that are part of a larger goal.

You'll also want to identify the resources you need to reach this goal. What human, material, and community resources do you have? Which of these will help you meet your goal? Plan to put these resources to their best use. Identify other uses of your resources that might conflict with your goal. Decide how you will limit or avoid these.

The next step in goal-setting is to put your plan into action. This is the step where you work toward achieving the goal. Keep track of your progress. If you fall short one day, don't give up. Forgive yourself and try to get back on track.

Getting Specific

General	Specific
to be a better student	to study for two hours each night this week
to raise my algebra grade	to earn at least a B on the next test
to get along with my parents	to communicate more clearly with my parents to reduce the chance of a fight this week
to be a better parent	to take a parenting class to learn more parenting skills
to keep my room clean	to put all my dirty clothes in the hamper and put all clean clothes away next time
to be a better friend	to keep all my plans with friends this month instead of canceling at the last minute
to get in shape	to jog half a mile every day for the next three weeks
to eat healthier	to eat at least three servings of vegetables each day this month and limit myself to one junk food "treat" a week
to improve my looks	to put on makeup, wear jewelry, and style my hair every day this month

3-7 By turning general goal statements into specific ones, you make your goals more measurable and easier to achieve.

It might also help to set small rewards for each subgoal you achieve. This will motivate you to keep working toward your main goal. You might also choose a reward for yourself when you achieve the main goal. Perhaps that reward could be enjoying your walk across the stage to receive your diploma at graduation. Whatever it is, the reward should mean something to you. It should be your special treat for achieving your goal.

Once you achieve your goal, you'll feel great! There is still one more thing to do, though. You need to evaluate the plan. What did you do right? What could you have done differently? If you were doing this again, how could you improve? Evaluating your efforts will help you learn what does and does not work well for you. This can make it easier to set future goals.

If you don't meet your goal, don't think of it as a failure. Use it as a learning experience. Modify your goal and try again. It may take some practice to set workable goals, but you can do it.

Decision Making

Part of becoming an adult is learning to make your own decisions. Some choices are difficult to make. Using a step-by-step process can make it a little easier. Take your time and carefully think through the decisions facing you. This will help you choose the best option. You'll also be less likely to regret your choices if you use the decision-making process. This process has six steps. See Figure 3-8. Each step is described in the paragraphs that follow. You will also read about a decision made by a teen parent named Loretta who used this process.

Identify the Decision to Be Made

In this step, you identify the choice to be made and commit to making a decision. Without a commitment, you are more likely to choose without thinking about the results. You might also give up if making a decision becomes hard. This first step is not very difficult, but it's important.

Chapter 3 Considering Values, Goals, and Decisions   63

Loretta had a dilemma. She was trying to decide whether to take a part-time job. Loretta loved her son, Mark, but having a child was expensive. She was tired of always having to ask her mother for the money to pay for baby items. Loretta had seen a "Help Wanted" sign in the window of the local grocery store. She knew the store's manager, Mr. Thomas. Loretta was sure he would hire her. All she had to do now was decide whether to apply for the job.

Gather and Examine Information

In this step, you will seek the information you need to make a wise decision. Learn all you can about the topic. One way to do this is by talking with people who know something about the choice you're facing. It may help to hear their experiences.

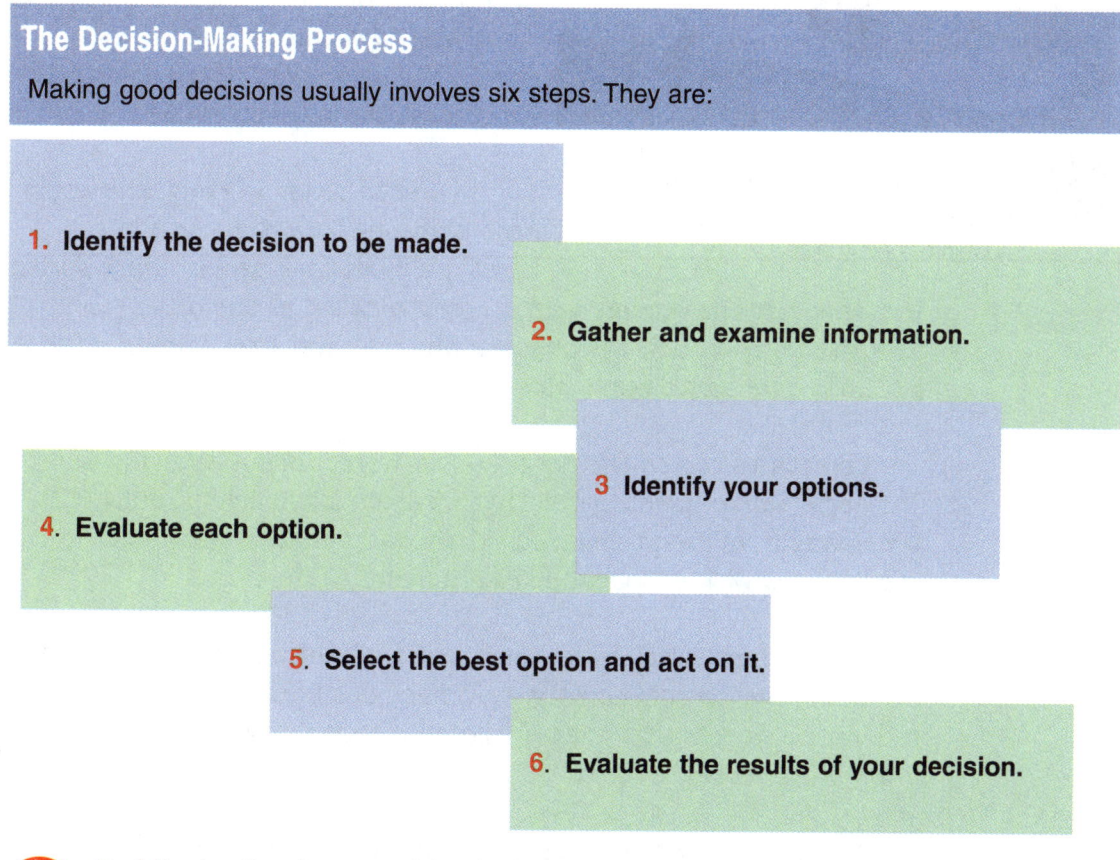

The Decision-Making Process
Making good decisions usually involves six steps. They are:

1. Identify the decision to be made.
2. Gather and examine information.
3. Identify your options.
4. Evaluate each option.
5. Select the best option and act on it.
6. Evaluate the results of your decision.

3-8 By following the six steps of the decision-making process, you can carefully arrive at the best decision for you.

Research can also help you gain information. Look for books, brochures, or magazine articles on the topic. Do an Internet search to learn more. See Figure 3-9. Perhaps you can interview someone in a career related to your decision. This may give you other information you need.

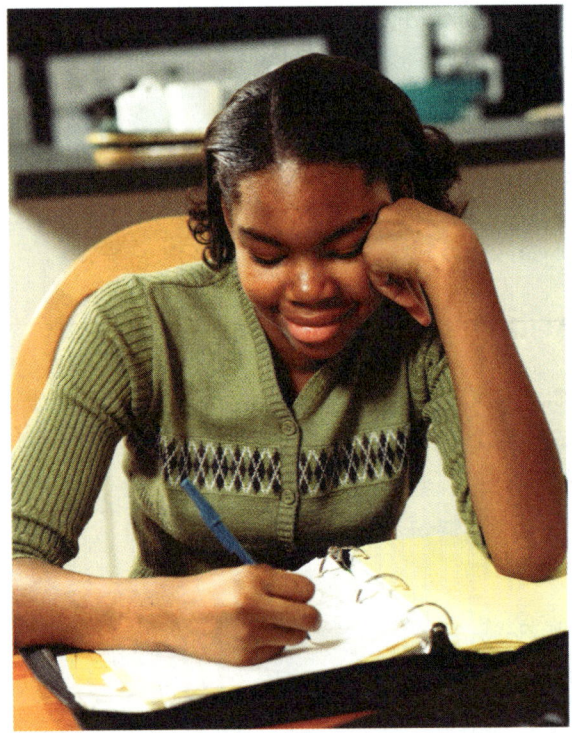

3-9 Get online to find out more about the issues involved with the decision you're making. This can help you make the most informed choice.

Loretta started to gather information related to the decision. She stopped by the grocery store for an application. Attached to the application was a sheet describing the job duties and expectations. From this sheet, she learned the hours of the job were 5 p.m. to 7 p.m. weekdays and one Saturday a month. This gave Loretta more information about what the job would involve.

If Loretta began working, she would need someone to watch her son. Loretta's mom took care of Mark during the week, but she worked nights. Loretta called all the other babysitters she knew. The only one who was available charged quite a bit. Child care costs would be expensive!

Loretta talked to the school social worker about this decision. The social worker pointed out that having a job is helpful, but it takes time away from everything else. At times, Loretta already felt overwhelmed with school and being a mom.

Later, Loretta talked to her friend, Samantha, who worked at the store. Samantha told Loretta how much she liked the job and what nice people worked at the store. Loretta thought they sounded like interesting people to meet.

Now Loretta felt she had the information she needed. She still felt confused about her choices, though. She wanted to take the job, but she knew it wouldn't be easy.

Identify Your Options

In this third step, you will brainstorm all the possible options you have regarding this decision. Now is not the time to judge the options; that will come later. You're just trying to determine what options are available. You may find it very helpful to list each option on a sheet of paper. This will prevent you from forgetting any of the options.

Loretta felt her choices were simple—either she would take the job or she would not. If she took the job, she would have to pay child care costs. She could ask her mom to watch Mark for the one Saturday each month the job required. Loretta could not identify any other options regarding this decision.

Evaluate Each Option

In this step, you will evaluate each option for its ability to work for you. You are trying to narrow your options by thinking more about each one.

Start by listing the pros and cons of each option. See Figure 3-10. These may be more obvious for some options than for others. Think about the good and bad sides of each available choice. The possible results of a decision are called consequences. Some of these can be positive, while others are negative. A wise decision has consequences that benefit you. Poor decisions often have harmful results. Look at both the short- and long-term consequences of an option. Even if the short-term benefits of an option are appealing, the long-term effects may not seem as good.

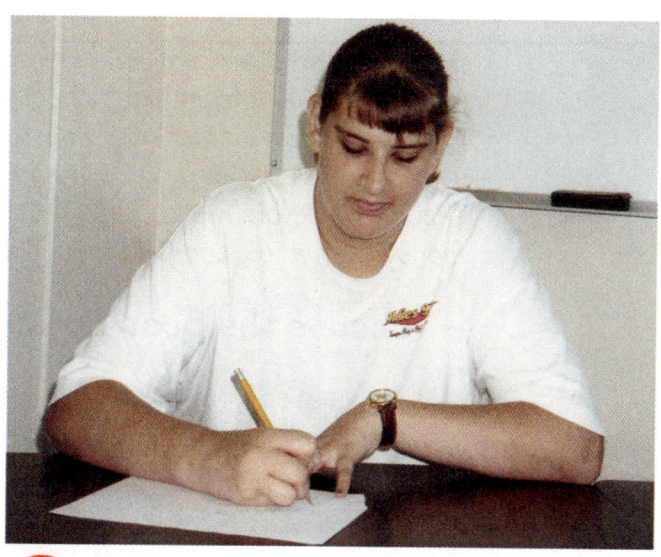

3-10 Writing a list of advantages and disadvantages can help you explore your options.

If you choose an option, you must be willing to accept the consequences that come with it. What if an option has consequences you're not willing to bear? Eliminate this choice from your list. This is not an option that will work well for you.

Finally, think about how your goals and values relate to this decision. Make a choice that will fit well with your goals and values. An option that interferes with them can cause you unneeded stress. You may want to remove from your list any options that compete with your goals and values.

Loretta listed both the advantages and disadvantages of taking the job. The biggest benefit would be earning the extra money. Other advantages included building her resume and learning some basic job skills. Working would have some disadvantages, too. The job would take even more time away from her child. Next were the added babysitting costs. Loretta would make about $80 a week, half of which would go to the babysitter. Having a job would also take time away from her studies and spending time with friends. Instead, she would take on even more responsibilities that might make her feel more overwhelmed.

Next, Loretta examined her goals and values. One of her goals was to graduate from high school with good enough grades to get into college. Her career goal was to become a food scientist. Loretta valued her education and her relationship with her son above all else. These values told her to pass up the job. Yet she needed the extra money from a job, too. This would help her take care of her son.

Choose the Best Option and Act on It

In this step, you make a final decision based on all the options you haven't eliminated. You choose the one you think will work best for you. Accept responsibility for your choice. Don't worry any more about whether this is the right decision—the choice is already made.

Now that you have made your decision, it's time to act on it. Follow through with the choice you've made. Be confident in your ability to make a good decision.

Suddenly, it seemed clear to Loretta she shouldn't take the job. It would be just too big a time commitment, and the financial costs were too high. Loretta decided this wasn't the job for her. Perhaps she'd find another job that would work better for her. Until then, Loretta would stay at home with Mark in the evenings.

Evaluate the Results of Your Decision

In this step, you are looking back on the decision you made. Did you make the right choice? Only after you have made a decision and carried it through do you really know if it was a good choice. Review your decision and think about what you might do differently next time. What did you learn from this process? See Figure 3-11.

If your decision didn't turn out exactly how you thought it would, you may be able to make some changes. This could make your decision fit you better. Sometimes this isn't possible, though.

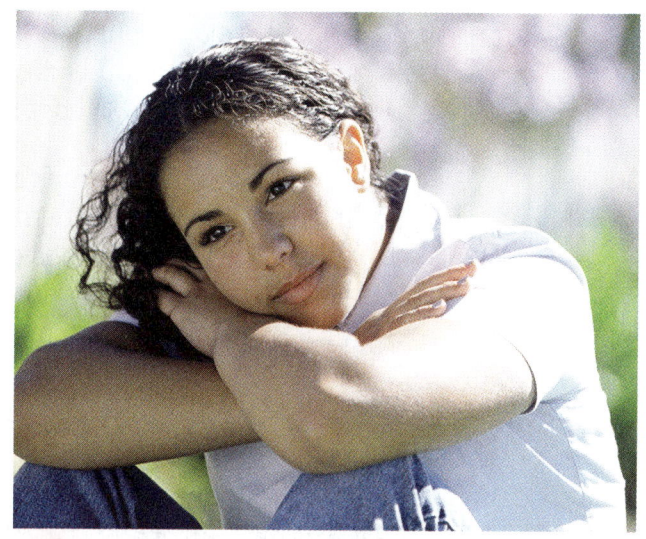

3-11 Take some time to reflect on the choice you have made. As you evaluate your decision, what have you learned?

Even if you decide this wasn't the best decision, it was the one you made. Accept responsibility for your choice. Don't blame anyone else or spend time wishing things were different. Learn from the experience and move on. Don't lose confidence—the next time things will likely work out better.

About a month later, Loretta decided to evaluate her decision. She felt she had made the best decision for her. She couldn't afford to work, given the cost of the babysitter and the time it would take away from her child and her studies. Loretta decided to wait until she graduated to look for a job again.

From Loretta's example, you can see how the decision-making process works. You can also see why it's useful. This process can help you arrive at the decision that will work best for you. If you carefully follow the steps, you can be sure you have thought of all the important aspects of the decision at hand.

Now you understand what values, goals, and resources are. You have learned how these important concepts relate to decision making. By using the decision-making process, you can carefully think through the decisions you face. Take your time to make important decisions. This will help you arrive at the best decision possible. Each good decision you make will boost your self-esteem.

Major Points

- Values are feelings, beliefs, and ideas about what is important. Your values will guide your behavior, goals, and decisions. Values are developed first by family. They are later influenced by friends, media, religious beliefs, and school. Personal experiences and choices play a role, too.

- A value conflict describes the tension caused by competing values or sets of values. Value conflicts can occur within a person or between people. Compromising and prioritizing are two ways to solve value conflicts.

- Values can be changed by the influences that shape them. You can change your values on your own. This involves identifying the change to make, reviewing your present values, and setting new priorities. Finally, bring your actions into line with your new values.

- Goals are statements of what you want to achieve. You can have both long-term and short-term goals. These goals are easiest to reach if they relate to your values.

- Resources are the means you use for accomplishing your goals. Three types include human, material, and community resources. Each type can help you reach your goals.

- Goal-setting involves several steps. These are stating the proposed goal, clarifying your goal, planning how to reach your goal, identifying resources, putting your plan into action, rewarding yourself, and evaluating your progress.

- The decision-making process provides a way to think through important decisions. Following this six-step process can help you make the decision that's best for you.

Chapter 4
Is Marriage in the Picture?

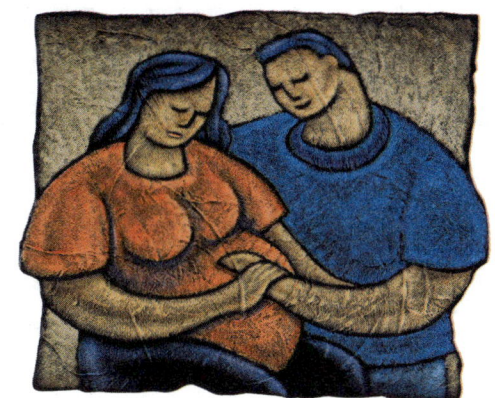

As you make choices about your pregnancy, you will think about many options. One of these may be marriage. Marriage is the emotional and legal commitment a man and woman make to become husband and wife. It is the declaration of a couple's wish to blend into one family unit. Marriage is generally thought of as a lifetime commitment. It is meant to last forever. Marriage can bring great joy, but it also takes work.

Your decision about marriage is a big one. It will take some time and a lot of thought. Marrying would change your life in many ways. You might not even be able to foresee all these ways. It might help to learn more about why teens marry and what is known about these marriages. This chapter also explains how marital roles have changed over time and how couples adjust to being married. It describes factors to think about when making this choice.

What Is Love?

Ask couples of any age why they married. The first answer given is usually love. People marry because they want to spend their lives together. For some couples, this love lasts a lifetime, with as many as 75 years of marriage.

For others, what they call love doesn't seem to last a month. Chances are, what these couples thought was love was really infatuation. This is an intense feeling of attraction that begins quickly and fades over time. People often confuse it with love, but the two are quite different. See Figure 4-1.

Is It Love?

Love differs from infatuation in many ways. These can be grouped into four main characteristics. A relationship based on love is each of the following:

✤ **Realistic**
each person understands, accepts, and appreciates the other

✤ **Steady and lasting**
each person's warm and tender feelings for the other build slowly and deepen over time

✤ **Caring**
each person supports and encourages the other; seeks what is best for the partner and the relationship as well as what is best for himself or herself

✤ **Mutually giving**
each person shows effort in the relationship and is concerned about the other's feelings

4-1 Does your relationship have the characteristics of love?

Infatuation is selfish. It causes you to focus on feeling good rather than on what the other person wants and needs. Strong, instant feelings of sexual desire are a part of infatuation. A person may feel led to act on these intense feelings without thinking about what is best for both people or the relationship. This selfish attitude can poison the relationship. It can leave one person feeling used when it ends.

On the other hand, love is a strong feeling of attachment, warmth, and understanding between two people. It is a steady, long-lasting feeling that builds slowly over time. Love can begin only when you truly get to know someone. Only then can you accept a person as he or she is, flaws included.

When people love each other, each truly cares about the other and has the other person's well-being as a high priority. They may also start to have sexual feelings for one another. Each person may think about showing his or her feelings in a physical way. This doesn't mean they act on those feelings, though. People who love each other think things through and take their time. They don't rush into anything. Each person wants what is best for both people and the relationship. They will wait to enter a sexual relationship until the time is right. If they are committed to spending their lives together, they know a sexual relationship will be most satisfying within the context of marriage.

In a marriage, love inspires each person to make the effort to keep the relationship strong. See Figure 4-2. In hard times, couples may feel fewer of the wonderful feelings that brought them together. At these times, commitment to the relationship can keep the marriage together until better times return.

Taking your time in a relationship will help you learn if your feelings are infatuation or love. Getting to know the other person will tell you a lot, too. Can you see your partner's faults? Do you accept and care about the total person? Pay attention to how he seems to feel about you as well. Make sure he treats you in a way that shows love rather than infatuation. A marriage based on infatuation is not likely to last, but one that is rooted in love is.

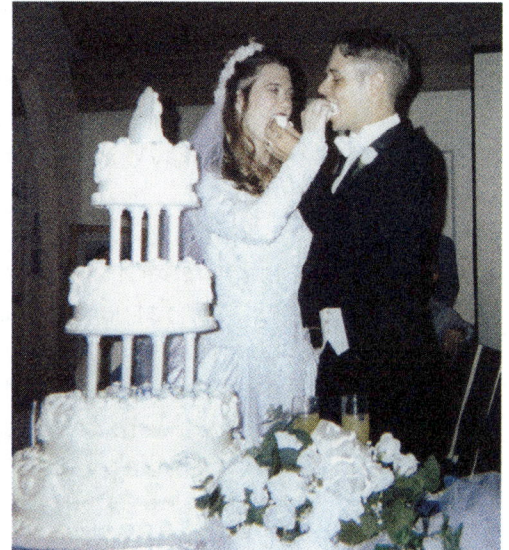

4-2 Love is important, but it's not the only component of a strong marriage.

Other Reasons Teens Marry

For what reasons other than love might teens marry? Several common reasons are described in the paragraphs that follow. Some are healthy reasons to marry, while others are less healthy. In many cases, more than one reason might be present.

Pregnancy

Marriage in the teen years is less common than it once was. Long ago, many people married in the teen years. Back then, many families farmed, while few people went to college or worked outside the home.

Today, most young people delay marriage until their middle or late twenties. Often, they want to complete their education and start a career before focusing on marriage.

Many of today's teen marriages happen as a result of pregnancy. When a young woman learns she is pregnant, she may think about marriage. This would give the child a two-parent family. It would also establish the teen parents as life partners. For these reasons, young couples may consider marriage if pregnancy occurs.

Today, fewer teens marry because of pregnancy than in the past. Young, unmarried women who became pregnant were once expected to marry the fathers or plan adoptions for their babies. These were the only options that were seen as acceptable. In the past, becoming an unmarried single parent was not considered an option. Forced teen marriages were called *shotgun weddings*. This phrase reflected the idea of a bride's father using a gun to force the young man to marry his pregnant daughter. You might also have heard the phrase "they had to get married" used to describe these marriages. Some young couples still feel pressured to marry when pregnancy occurs, but this happens far less often today.

A marriage has the best chance when both partners love one another and are committed to the relationship. If the relationship is already strong, it is more likely to hold up under the pressures of marriage and parenting. In this situation, the couple can work together to adjust to the changes. If a couple is willing to put in the effort a strong marriage requires, this type of marriage can be successful.

Marriages are less likely to last when the couple marries "for the baby's sake." If the child is the couple's main reason for being married, the marriage may suffer. Having a baby will not strengthen a weak relationship. Instead, the marriage may crack under the pressures of marriage and parenting.

To Cure Loneliness

Some teens may marry for fear of being alone. Teens who lack self-esteem may find it hard to believe anyone would want to marry them. They may think this partner is their one and only chance to marry. These teens might marry without thinking about whether it is the right time or the right person. Teens, however, have many years ahead of them to meet the right mate and marry. Being patient and believing in themselves can help them wait until the time is right.

Other people marry because they feel lonely. They want to escape these feelings of loneliness. These people may assume the other person will meet their needs for constant company. Marriage, they might think, means being together all the time. Actually, even married people need some time and space of their own. Otherwise they can start to feel smothered. Each partner needs time to pursue personal interests. See Figure 4-3. This makes the marriage stronger.

It is not a good idea to marry out of loneliness. People who do this soon learn the other person cannot make them happy. The satisfaction they seek must come from within themselves. A marriage that happens for this reason can become strained. One partner feels smothered and the other keeps feeling lonely. Over time, the strain can cause the marriage to end.

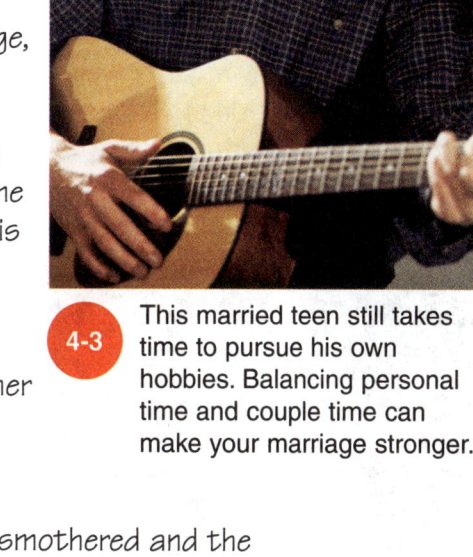

4-3 This married teen still takes time to pursue his own hobbies. Balancing personal time and couple time can make your marriage stronger.

To Make Them Feel Complete

Some teens may marry because they think it will help them feel fulfilled and complete. Such a person may feel he or she has something missing inside. The person may seek marriage hoping the other person can fill this empty space.

Often, this type of marriage soon falls apart. One partner keeps asking more of the other. The other partner becomes frustrated because he or she can never give enough to please this person. He or she may soon feel taken advantage of and tired of trying. This relationship isn't satisfying for either partner.

Each person should be a complete, whole person on his or her own. This will help the marriage succeed. If you feel incomplete, try to discover why you feel this way. Work to find happiness and fulfillment in yourself as a person before you marry. This will give you a healthier start when you do marry.

To Escape Unhappy Home Lives

Some teens feel unhappy living at home with their parents. Abuse or mistreatment may be common in these homes. Teens may resent always being told what to do by their parents. They may see marriage as the only way to escape their home lives. It may seem living on their own and making their own decisions will make them happier. Being "rescued" from their current situations by their partners may seem ideal.

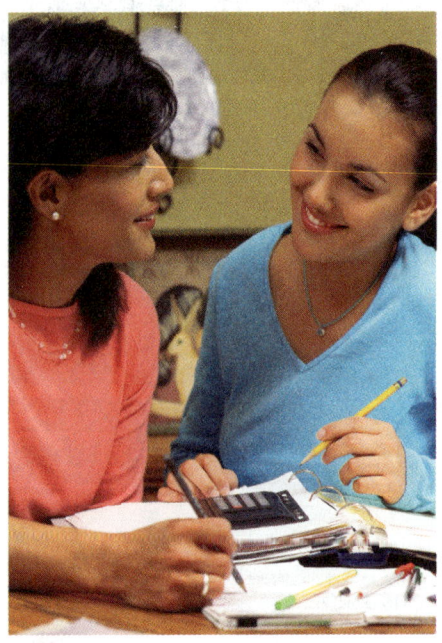

4-4 A part-time job helps, but it won't supply all the income a teen couple needs to live on their own and raise their child.

In reality, though, things don't usually work out this well. Many teens may discover marriage brings less freedom than they had hoped. Even when people live on their own, they still have many rules to follow. For instance, they have laws to obey, contracts to fulfill (such as leases), bills to pay, and supervisors at work to whom they must answer. On their own, they also have many more responsibilities. Managing money is tough, especially for teens who don't have full-time jobs. Most teens work a few hours a week at fairly low wages. See Figure 4-4. In this case, teen couples may not be able to make enough money to live on their own. Couples who married to escape home often end up moving back to their parents' homes for financial reasons.

Rather than marrying to escape home, it's wiser to seek help with the problems occurring there. Counseling may help you identify problems and decide how to handle them. It can also help you resolve feelings about what has been happening at home. If you're being abused or mistreated at home, talk with a trusted adult. This person can help you. You need a safe home environment in which to live, especially if you are bringing a baby into it.

To Gain Money or Social Status

Have you ever heard of someone who married to gain money or social status? This kind of person tries to use marriage to secure a better position in life. He or she desires the partner's lifestyle, but doesn't really love the partner. This person may soon find he or she is unhappy. No amount of money can buy happiness. Being married to someone you don't love can be difficult. It doesn't bring the kind of joy you will find if you marry someone you truly love. Also, marriage requires both partners to give and take. Without a strong motivation of love, people generally won't continue giving in a one-sided fashion over time.

To Become Life Partners

Teens may also want to marry to become life partners. Marriage makes them a family. These teens are often emotionally mature. They are committed to each other and their relationship. These are the most healthy marriages and the most likely to last. See Figure 4-5.

This kind of couple is able to talk through problems and express their feelings. Neither partner is selfish—each strives to meet the other's needs. Each spouse loves the other deeply and cares about the spouse's well-being. Both are willing to give the time and effort their marriage needs. Their relationship is mutual, or two-sided. It involves give and take on both sides.

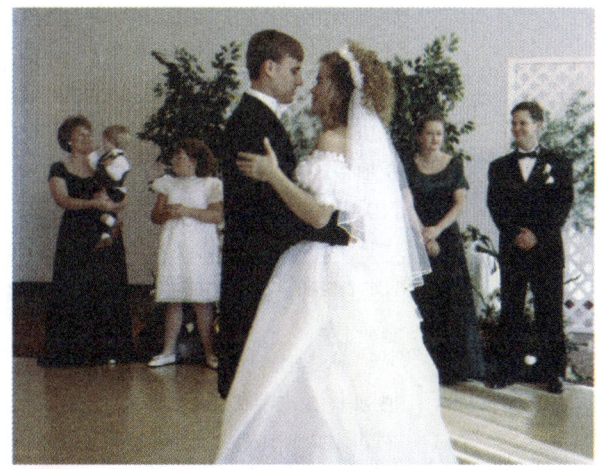

4-5 Marriages based on partnership are often the most successful.

This type of marriage is the best for parenting. It's good for children when both parents love and respect each other. These parents set a good example for their children. They can also offer the children a stable home life. A parent with a committed partner also feels less stress. This is because both parents can share the responsibilities and decisions.

Why Do Some Teen Marriages Fail?

When they marry, most couples want to be happy and stay married forever. Yet today almost half of all marriages end in divorce. This figure is even higher for teen marriages, with only 4 out of 10 lasting. About 60 percent of married teens separate or divorce within five years.

Why do so many teen marriages end in divorce? There can be many reasons for this. First, some people have unrealistic expectations of marriage. They hope being married will solve all their problems—but it doesn't. Marriage can even make some problems worse.

Lack of commitment can also break up teen marriages. A marriage won't succeed unless both partners are devoted to making it work. This takes effort and patience. For many, being married is harder than they imagined. Some teens aren't willing to give this much to their relationships. Others find they really weren't ready to commit. They may feel they've missed much of what life has to offer. No matter the reason, a lack of commitment can cause problems. If one partner gives more than the other, he or she may soon feel taken for granted. This can cause unhappiness and may lead to divorce.

A lack of maturity may also lead teen marriages to end. Marriage is difficult at times for adults. It is even harder for teens, who are still forming their identities. In general, the younger a person is at marriage, the more likely it is that divorce will occur. This means someone who marries at age 16 is more likely to divorce than someone who marries at age 20. Much of this is due to changes a person experiences in the teen years. Some of these changes can cause a couple to grow apart, making divorce more likely.

People's interests may also change as they mature. They may not enjoy doing the same things or being with the same people as before. A couple may grow apart and share less in common than before. Each person may become attracted to someone else with more similar interests. This can lead couples to end their marriages.

What else is known about teens who marry? Married teens are more likely to struggle with finances than couples who marry later. This is especially true if they quit school. Without at least a high school diploma, there are few jobs that pay well. Without education or experience, they are not likely to make enough money to support themselves. See Figure 4-6.

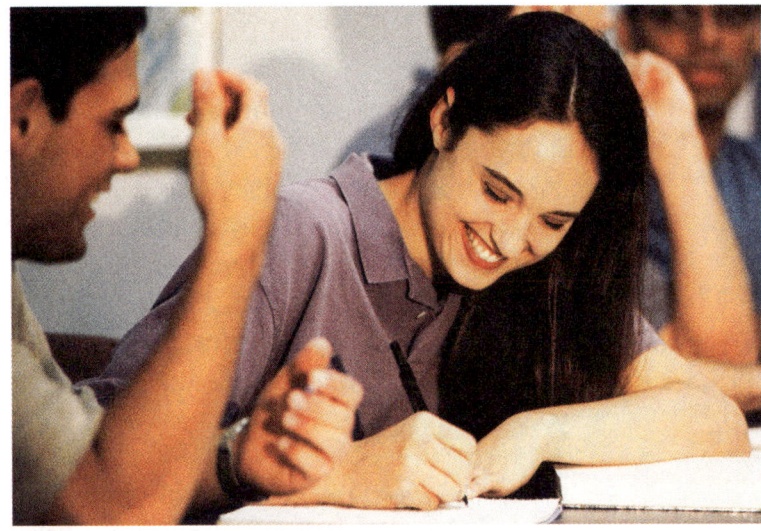

4-6 Education is important, even for married teens. Finishing school can allow you and your spouse to find jobs that can support your family.

Couples who marry in their teens are also more likely to live with one spouse's parents than those who marry later. Many teen couples cannot afford to live on their own. Even if they married to escape home, money matters may keep them there. They may feel trapped, living with their parents only to avoid being homeless. This unhappiness can put strain on a marriage.

Living with parents can help teen couples lower their expenses. It can also be a big adjustment. With more people in the house, disputes over everyday living issues can arise. The new member of the household may have trouble fitting into the style and routine of the partner's family. This can cause stress. If the in-laws don't approve of the marriage or their teen's mate, this can make things even harder. Finally, problems can arise if the teen couple's parents disagree with how the couple parents their child. It takes a strong marriage to overcome these problems and stresses.

Despite the odds, some teen marriages last. In these relationships, each partner is committed to the other and the marriage. These couples work hard to overcome the struggles and problems that occur. Hard times help the spouses mature and grow closer. These couples put in the effort needed to keep their marriages strong. The happiness and comfort that marriage brings them lasts a lifetime.

How Are Marital Roles Changing?

As you consider marriage, it's good to think about what your role and your partner's role would be. A role is a set of behaviors that is linked to a certain position you fill in life. Right now, some of your roles may include daughter, sister, aunt, student, and employee. Being a parent is another role. If you decide to marry, you will add the role of spouse. What actions will change as you and your partner become spouses? How will you interact with each other and manage family matters? In answering these questions, the two of you are setting your marital roles.

In the past, only one set of marital roles was accepted by society. Almost all married couples followed these roles. Now, however, things are changing. Today, couples can work together to define what their marital roles will be.

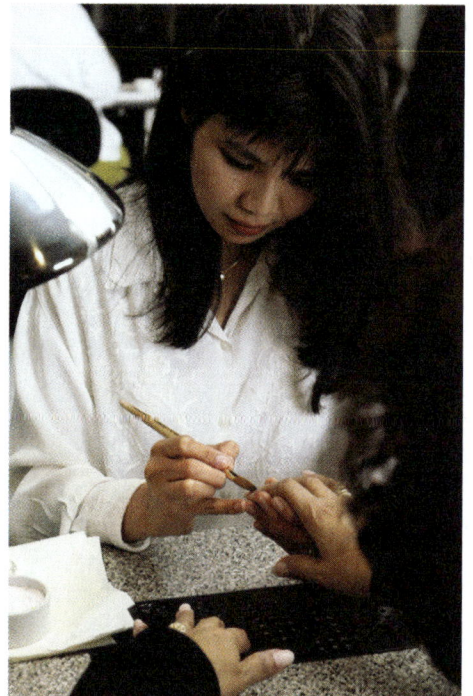

4-7 This woman splits the task of earning money for the family with her husband. They share other roles, too.

For many years, the husband's role in the family was to be the provider, or wage earner. He was responsible for earning money to support his family. This may have been by growing crops. It could also have been by working outside the home. The man also handled the family's budget, purchases, and decision making.

In this family, the wife's role was to be the supporter of her family. She maintained the home and its resources. She did tasks such as cooking, cleaning, and sewing. The wife also had the primary job of raising the children.

Today, some families still follow this pattern. Most, however, do not. Now many wives work outside the home. See Figure 4-7. A family in which both parents work outside the home is called a dual-career family. In these families, spouses often split housework and parenting tasks more evenly. Since both parents work, neither has the energy to do it all alone. These couples often define their roles based on what will work best for their situation. In these families, wives might mow the lawn and husbands might put the children to bed.

Before you marry, think about the roles you expect yourself and your partner to play. Talk with your partner about this. Are his ideas similar to yours? Can the two of you compromise in areas where you disagree? If not, you may wish to reconsider marriage. When partners have conflicting expectations about what their roles will be, it can cause problems in the marriage.

How Do Couples Adjust to Marriage?

You will face adjustments every time a major change occurs in your life. When many changes occur at once, you'll have even more adjustments to make. This is one reason it's harder to be married as a teen than as an adult. The teen years themselves are a time of great change. Suppose you add the new roles of parent and spouse. By themselves, each of these adjustments can be difficult. Handling them all at once is much more challenging.

As couples adjust to marriage and parenting, the partners won't always agree. This is normal. All couples have some conflicts. How the partners work together to handle these conflicts can affect how happy the marriage is. If they can talk things out, they'll be able to resolve these conflicts and enjoy marriage. Otherwise, minor conflicts can turn into major problems. This could cause the spouses to have a harder time getting along.

Many of these adjustments relate to living together. Spouses may differ in their routines, housekeeping, and preferences. Even simple issues can cause a disagreement. Two people may not like the same toothpaste or TV shows. These issues don't matter much in the big picture of life. Always arguing over small things can take some of the joy out of their marriage. It may also mean larger fights over more important issues.

To preserve their marriage, both partners must communicate. Each person can give in and handle some matters in the other person's way. It's also good to keep minor household issues in perspective. Many disputes really aren't worth the problems they cause. In time, each partner will get used to the other's way of doing things. This is part of learning how to live together.

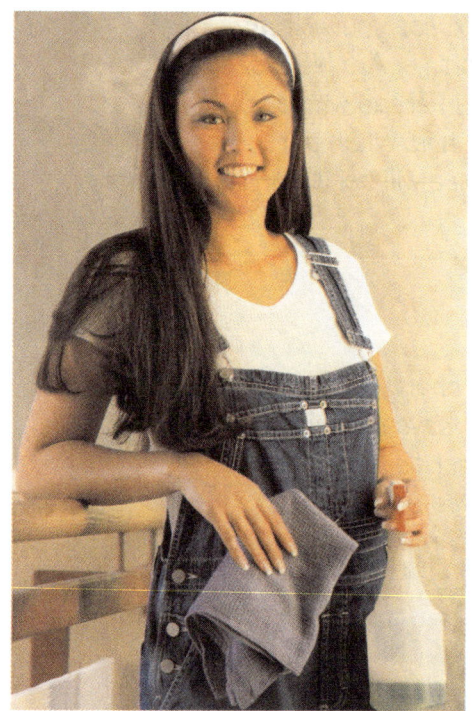

4-8 In addition to school, work, and parenting, married teens also have housekeeping and other home maintenance tasks to complete.

When a person marries, he or she also takes on the role of daughter- or son-in-law. This role can be fairly easy to adopt or it may be tough. This depends mostly on how well the person gets along with the in-laws. Some in-laws are easy to please and accept their child's new spouse quickly. These in-laws can share their knowledge and help the young couple in many ways. Other in-laws do not adjust as easily. They may dislike the situation and take it out on their child's new spouse. Living with these in-laws can be a challenge. When this happens, it's best to simply try to get along.

Adjusting to parenthood also brings challenges for married teens. One or both spouses might have to work to earn income for the family. They may need to juggle a full schedule of work, school, parenting, and household chores. See Figure 4-8. This can be difficult if they get little sleep because they're up at night caring for a child. When both spouses share tasks, it can really help. Maybe partners can take turns getting up at night with the baby. Both can handle chores around the house, too. It can help when both spouses can talk clearly about their needs and expectations.

Examining Your Situation

One of the big choices you may make during your pregnancy is whether to marry. For some the answer is clear; others have a harder time deciding. Each person's situation is unique. What's best for one person may not be right for you. As you decide, you may wish to think about the questions on the next page.

Chapter 4   Is Marriage in the Picture?

- 👉 Is marriage an option for you right now?
- 👉 Is your partner the right person for you to marry?
- 👉 Are you ready to marry?
- 👉 What might happen if you waited to marry?

Is Marriage an Option Right Now?

The first question to consider is whether marrying is an option for you at this time. In some cases, it may not be. There can be many reasons for this. Some of these include the following:

- 👉 You and the baby's father were not in a serious relationship when the pregnancy occurred. The two of you may have dated casually. You may not have known each other well or thought of him as a future spouse. It could be you were no longer in contact with him when you learned of your pregnancy.

- 👉 You and the baby's father ended your relationship after the pregnancy began. The two of you may have broken up since you learned of your pregnancy. You may have decided you were a poor match. He may have left you rather than accept his responsibilities as a father. You may not even be in contact with him anymore.

- 👉 The baby's father (or your current partner) is not interested in marrying you. Suppose you want to get married and, for whatever reason, the other person doesn't. This can be hard to accept. If that's how he feels, though, it's probably best not to marry. One or both of you would likely be very unhappily married.

- 👉 You don't want to marry the baby's father (or your current partner). Even if he asked you to marry him, you might say no. You may not be ready or think he is the right person. Instead, you might want to focus on other goals. These might be completing school and preparing to be a parent. Perhaps the relationship isn't serious enough to think about marriage right now.

- 👉 The baby's father (or your current partner) abuses you or is involved in illegal activities. Neither of these types of partners is safe to marry. You cannot change this person or his dangerous behavior. It is best to leave this type of relationship at once.

A partner's illegal activities can have negative results for you. In some cases, it may be illegal to know about a crime without stopping it or contacting the police. You might also be arrested for a crime you didn't commit. It is wise not to marry this type of person. You and your child deserve a better, safer life.

If your partner is abusive, it is also safest to leave the relationship as soon as you can. Marriage almost always makes abuse worse. Leaving may also be harder after you're married. You don't deserve to be abused, nor do you want your child to witness or suffer abuse. If you need help to leave, call a domestic violence hot line. They may be able to offer you a place to stay or ideas about how to leave safely. Counseling is also available at these agencies.

Is This the Right Person for You?

Before you marry, you want to be sure you have chosen a person who will be a good match for you. This is essential. Would the person you're considering make a good spouse and a good parent?

What qualities do you think are important in a spouse? See Figure 4-9. What people look for in a mate differs somewhat from person to person. There are a few basic qualities that are almost always important, though. Some of these include the following:

- Good communication skills. This means being able to talk to others and listen to them. Communication should not be one-sided. It is an active process that involves two people. Expressing your thoughts and feelings can bring you closer to your mate. Choose a spouse who can communicate well, too.

- Personality traits. Do you like being with your potential spouse and having fun together? If being with this person often annoys you, this is a danger sign. After marriage, annoying traits can turn into major issues. Realize you can never change anyone but yourself. For this reason, be sure you genuinely like the person you've chosen <u>before</u> you marry.

- Grooming and hygiene. Most people hope for an attractive spouse. For many, however, good looks aren't the top priority. Good hygiene (personal cleanliness) habits and a desire to take care of oneself matter, too. Have you ever known a

What Do You Want in a Mate?

Read each of the following descriptions. For each, check the appropriate response. How important is it for your future mate to be...

	Very Important	Important	Unimportant	Very Unimportant
1. affectionate				
2. understanding				
3. honest				
4. faithful				
5. humorous				
6. concerned about others				
7. attractive in appearance				
8. pleasant in personality				
9. positive in outlook				
10. hard-working				
11. well-educated				
12. emotionally mature				
13. self-confident				
14. a good communicator				
15. accepting of constructive criticism				
16. responsible with money				
17. wealthy				
18. good with children				
19. similar to you in background				
20. similar to you in interests				

4-9 Use this checklist to help you think about what qualities you want in a mate.

good-looking person who didn't take care of himself or herself? If so, how did this affect the person's looks? Grooming and hygiene can help all people look their best.

☛ Faithfulness. Most people want a spouse who will be faithful. This means neither spouse will have sex outside the marriage. Faithfulness can give you a sense of security and trust. It allows you to share with your partner in a safe, open way.

- Similarities. Do you want a spouse who is like you in some ways? Many people do. Some ways you might want your spouse to be like you include interests, culture, background, and religious beliefs. You might also want a spouse who has reached or is working toward the same level of education as you have.

- Financial responsibility. Most people want a mate who is responsible with money and can manage it wisely. This person is not wasteful. One or both spouses must be able to make enough money to support the family. Couples should decide who will work and who will care for their children. Talk about this before marriage to ensure you have chosen a mate who feels as you do.

Are You Ready to Marry?

Before you marry, you need to be sure you're ready. Marriages need time, effort, and nurturing to stay strong. Can you give this to your spouse, or are you more focused on other things in your life right now?

Take some time to determine whether marrying right now is best for you and your partner. Rushing into a marriage usually leads to feeling it was a mistake. This is why you need to be sure before you commit.

The following five factors have been found to show a readiness for marriage:

- Maturity and responsibility. A good marriage partner is responsible and mature. When you marry, you leave your childhood behind. You will take on more adult roles and responsibilities. You and your spouse will work together to head a family. This is a big job.

- Commitment to personal growth. This refers to your plans to better yourself as a person. A good spouse knows it's important to keep growing as a person. Learning more or improving your skills will enhance your life and your marriage.

- Emotional openness. If you have this quality, you are able to express your feelings easily with your partner. You are also able to hear his point of view. This aspect of communication and caring is vital to a happy marriage.

- Honesty. Honesty means being truthful. A good marriage partner is honest with his or her spouse even when it's easier to lie. This doesn't mean being cruel or hurtful—it merely means telling the truth. Honesty is doing what is right because you want to, not because you're forced.

- Self-esteem. To be a good marriage partner, you need to have self-esteem. This means you respect yourself and care about how others treat you. Liking yourself as a person gives you a sense of confidence and peace. It can also give you a positive outlook. These are desirable qualities to bring to a marriage.

Take a moment to think about how you rate in each area. This should give you an idea whether you're ready for marriage. You can also use the questions in Figure 4-10. Finally, you may want to set goals for yourself related to these areas. Achieving these goals can help you become a better person, no matter when you choose to marry.

Just as important is whether your spouse-to-be is ready for marriage. Talk with your partner about this issue. Based on what you know about your partner, do you think he is ready for marriage?

What About Waiting?

Many reasons might lead you to marry. Sometimes there are just as many (or more) reasons <u>not</u> to marry. In the end, only you can decide if marriage at this time is right for you.

Suppose you choose not to marry now. Accept your decision as the right one for you. Don't feel badly about yourself or regret your decision. Not marrying doesn't make you less of a person. In fact, it takes a strong person to know and admit that marrying right now isn't the right choice. This is better than marrying for the wrong reason and being unhappy later. You may wonder, however, what not marrying now means for you and your future.

Assessing Your Readiness for Marriage

Personal Growth
- What have I learned from past relationships and how will I use this to help me in my current relationship?
- Do I maintain important relationships besides the one I share with my partner?
- Do I have a balance between personal time and time with my partner? Do I pursue my own goals and interests?
- What are my greatest strengths and weaknesses? What am I doing to better myself?
- What changes would I like to see in myself five years from now? What habits would I like to eliminate or enhance?

Emotional Openness
- Can I recognize my emotions? Can I accept and control my feelings?
- Do I express my emotions in an appropriate way? Am I able to give and receive love freely?
- Can I share openly with my partner? Which emotions are difficult for me to talk about?
- Am I concerned about what is going on in my partner's life? Do I actively listen to my partner's feelings and concerns? Do I welcome him or her to share?

Honesty
- Do I have a history of being honest with others? How would my parents and my best friend rate me in terms of honesty? How would I rate myself?
- Do I know how to share the truth in a tactful way? Can I be honest even if it will hurt the other person's feelings?
- Have I cheated on my partner or kept secrets from him or her? Would I ever betray or lie to my partner?

Maturity and Responsibility
- Can I handle all the responsibility of marriage? Am I able to put the needs of my spouse and children ahead of my needs when necessary?
- Can I think issues through and decide what's best for me and my family?
- Do I accept my choices and their consequences without blaming others?
- Am I ready to commit to a lifelong relationship? Do I have realistic expectations of what marriage involves?
- In what areas of my life have I shown irresponsible behavior? Am I working to improve in these areas?
- Am I willing to give and take in solving problems?

Self-Esteem
- Do I depend upon another person to make me feel happy, loved, or worthwhile as a person?
- Is it important to me to respect myself and others? Do I seek positive relationships?
- Do I allow other people to take advantage of me?
- Do I feel complete as a person, with or without being married?

4-10 Are you ready for marriage? This list of questions can help you consider whether this is the right time for you to marry.

Not marrying now does <u>not</u> mean you and your partner can't stay together. The two of you can keep dating as long as you're both pleased with how the relationship is going. You can find other ways to be there for each other at this important time in your lives. Each of you can provide emotional support for the other. If you choose parenting, you and your partner can be there for your child even if you're not married. See Figure 4-11.

Delaying marriage does <u>not</u> mean you can't consider it again later. You can. As you and your partner grow closer, the two of you may discuss it again. At that time, you may be more ready for marriage. Your marriage will be more likely to last then, because the relationship is stronger.

Not marrying now does <u>not</u> mean you won't ever marry. You have many years ahead of you. Even if you parent, your chances of finding a mate in the future are high. By waiting for the right person and the right time, you can also increase the chance your marriage will be a success.

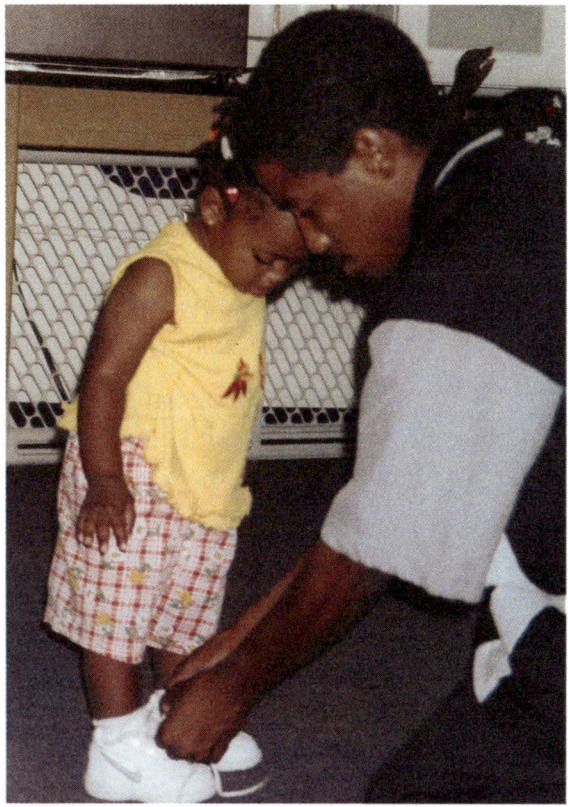

4-11 A father can choose to participate in his child's life no matter whether he's married to the child's mother.

Major Points

☛ Teens may choose to marry for many reasons; some are positive and others are less positive. These include pregnancy, to cure loneliness, to make them feel complete, to escape unhappy home lives, to gain money or social status, and to become life partners.

☛ Only about 4 in 10 teen marriages last more than five years. Teen marriages fail for a variety of reasons. Teens often have unrealistic expectations about marriage. They may lack the maturity and commitment marriage requires. Financial struggles and living with one of the teens' parents can cause problems, too.

- Marital roles have changed over the years. Traditionally, the only accepted marital roles were men as providers and women as supporters. Today's couples have more choices about the marital roles they will adopt.

- Newly married teens have many adjustments to make. These are learning to live with the other person (and often his or her parents), learning to juggle multiple roles, and learning to parent. Couples need patience, communication, and compromise to help them adjust.

- Your decision about marriage will be your own. As you decide, you may wish to consider whether marriage is an option for you right now. Have you found the right person, and are you ready for marriage? What would happen if you waited to marry?

Chapter 5
What Does It Mean to Be a Parent?

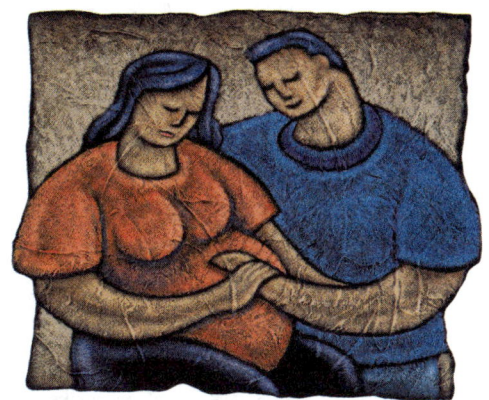

What is a parent? Is it simply a person who provides the sperm or egg to create a child? Yes, this person is technically a parent. A person can become a birthparent or biological parent through the birth of his or her child. Marriage and adoption are other ways to become a parent. A person who becomes a parent through marriage is a stepparent. An adoptive parent takes on the parenting role through the adoption process. Finally, a foster parent is an adult who serves as a parent by volunteering to provide a temporary home to a child in need of one.

The parenting role is more than just a title, though. A parent raises a child and provides for her total welfare. He or she gives the child daily care, love, support, and guidance. This person also works to meet the child's emotional, physical, social, and intellectual needs. Often, this responsibility lasts at least 18 years—from the time the child is born until she is legally an adult. Being a parent often means putting your own wants and needs aside. Your child's needs must be your first priority. One of her needs is to have a mature parent. This may mean you have to grow up fast.

Why should you learn about parenting? You have many decisions to make about your pregnancy. When you know what parenting involves, you can make an informed choice. In this chapter, you will learn about the responsibilities of parenting. You'll also learn why people choose to be or not to be parents. You can use what you've learned as you decide about parenthood.

If you choose to parent, you'll need to develop parenting skills. Many people think parenting is instinctive, or based on a natural skill or ability. They assume people know how to parent without being taught. While some parenting skills are instinctive, many are not. It takes patience and practice to learn new ways to guide and direct your child. You can learn these skills by taking a class or reading books on the subject. You have also learned from how your own parents raised you and how families close to you modeled parenting skills.

If you study parenting, it can have a good effect on your self-esteem. Learning more about children and how to guide them can boost your confidence. It can make you feel good about yourself and reassure you about what you're doing right. You can also learn new ways to solve problems with your child that might otherwise frustrate you. This, too, can make you feel more skilled as a parent. In turn, your increased self-esteem helps you view your role as a parent in a more positive way. It also sets a good example for your child as she develops her own self-esteem.

Parenting Responsibilities and Rewards

Each role you have brings with it a set of responsibilities. Being a parent is no exception. Parents have many responsibilities when it comes to raising their children. See Figure 5-1. Take a moment to think about each responsibility listed. Do you feel prepared to handle each of these duties? Can you think of any other responsibilities that parents have? What kind of training might prepare you for these tasks? Do you think you would have to learn as you went along? Handling these tasks takes practice.

Parenting also has many rewards. First and foremost, many people just enjoy being parents. They get satisfaction from this role. As a parent, you would have the reward of watching your child learn and grow. Giving to and caring for another person can be a good feeling. You would also have the joy of sharing your knowledge and time with your child. You would be there for all the special moments of his childhood. Parenting is hard work, but many parents feel it is well worth the effort. They find the joys they experience make up for the difficult times.

Chapter 5   What Does It Mean to Be a Parent?

> ### What Do Parents Do?
>
> Parents' responsibilities include the following:
> - providing financial support for their children
> - providing nutritious food, proper clothing, and adequate shelter for their children
> - offering love and emotional support to their children
> - monitoring their children's health and education
> - helping children meet their social and intellectual needs
> - guiding and disciplining their children appropriately at all ages
> - setting a good example for their children to follow
> - teaching their children about their heritage and culture
> - helping children learn responsibility, moral behavior, and family values
> - teaching children how to solve problems and make decisions
> - creating family routines that meet the needs of all family members
> - monitoring their children's growth and guiding their development

5-1 Are you prepared to handle all these parenting responsibilities? If not, how can you learn more?

To Parent or Not to Parent?

As you can see, parenting requires a lot from a person. Parenthood involves many adult responsibilities. It's a big job, often with little recognition. If parenting is so hard, you may wonder why people want to become parents. Figure 5-2 lists common reasons that people choose to parent or not to parent. There are many reasons a person might choose (or not choose) parenthood. Which of the reasons in the chart seem like good ones? Do some of the reasons seem immature? What are your reasons for choosing to parent or not to parent?

Some of the reasons given for becoming a parent are good ones. Good reasons focus on what the parent wants to do for the child. These reasons are better than those that focus on what the parent wants the child to do for him or her. A good reason is wanting to nurture and teach a child. This focuses on what you want to offer the child. A mature person who wants to meet a child's needs will usually be an effective parent. This person is dedicated to his or her children. He or she takes the time to guide their development.

Common Reasons for Parenting or Not Parenting

For Parenting	For Not Parenting
I feel a child will strengthen my relationship with my mate.	My relationship with my partner is not good enough for us to be parents.
I want to have a traditional family, and that lifestyle includes children.	I want my child to have two parents, and I cannot give him that right now.
I feel my life will be incomplete without having a child.	I didn't have good experiences as a child. I'm afraid I would not be good as a parent.
I want to share my love and knowledge with a child.	I am not mature enough to handle the responsibilities of parenting.
I want to nurture and teach a child.	I am devoted to pursuing career goals that are not compatible with parenting.
I want to experience the warm feelings having a child gives parents.	Children are expensive. I am not financially able to provide for a child.
I want someone to love me.	I value freedom. I am afraid children would be too confining.
I want a reason to leave home. Having a child will prove I am grown up.	I have health problems I don't want to pass on to a child.
I want to prove my femininity or masculinity.	I do not enjoy children and am not interested in being a parent.
I don't have a choice since I'm pregnant.	My partner doesn't want to parent, and I don't want to raise a child by myself.

5-2 Which of these reasons are good reasons for having or not having a child? Which ones reflect your own opinions?

Other reasons that people choose parenting seem illogical. These reasons are more focused on what the person hopes to gain from being a parent. They don't consider whether the person really wants to be a parent and care for a child. For instance, suppose a person envisions having a child as a way to gain love and acceptance. This person might think of a baby as someone to keep him or her company. These unrealistic expectations are unfair to the child.

When faced with a pregnancy, some teens choose not to become parents. These teens may not feel ready for this much work and responsibility. They may not feel they can give a child everything she needs. These teens may choose to pursue other goals at this time in their lives. To some, these reasons may seem selfish. In reality, it's wise for teens to realize if parenting is not for them. See Figure 5-3.

Factors to Consider

You have many factors to consider when deciding whether to become a parent. Each of these factors may affect your choice about becoming a parent right now.

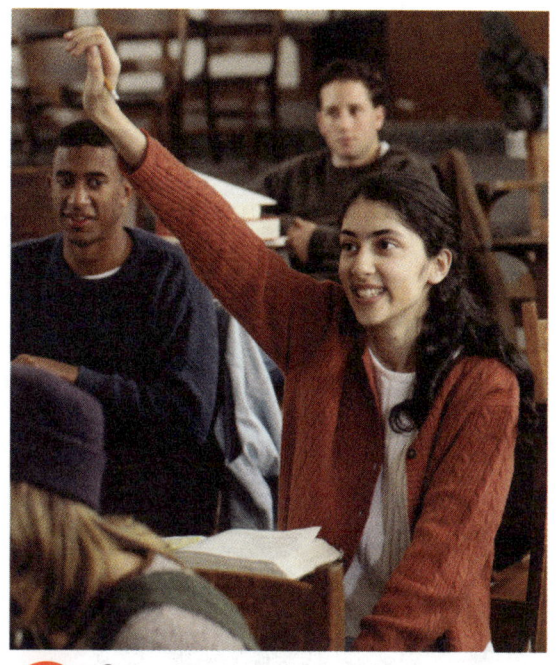

5-3 Some teens decide not to parent because they don't want to postpone their other goals. This young woman wants to go to college without delay so she can enter her chosen career.

Health

Before you become a parent, consider your health and that of your partner. First, are there any congenital disorders in your families? A congenital disorder is one that is inherited and is present from birth. Down syndrome and sickle cell anemia are two common congenital disorders. If any disorder runs in your family, you could pass it on to your child. You should think about what this might mean for the child's health. Both you and your partner can talk to your parents and grandparents about this. They are likely to know what disorders run in your family.

Also, are you healthy enough to withstand pregnancy and childbirth? (These events can be hard on a woman's body, and even more so if she's a teen.) After the baby arrives, parenting can take a toll on you. This job requires a lot of energy. Are you and the baby's father in good enough health to provide the care a child would need? Do either of you have chronic health problems? If so, how might this affect your ability to parent? You might also think about how parenting might affect your health.

Age

Age of the woman at pregnancy is also a factor. Teens have higher rates of health problems and complications related to pregnancy than women in their twenties. This is because a teen's body is not yet fully developed. A teen may also be less likely to take care of herself than a woman in her twenties. She may have poor eating, resting, and exercising habits.

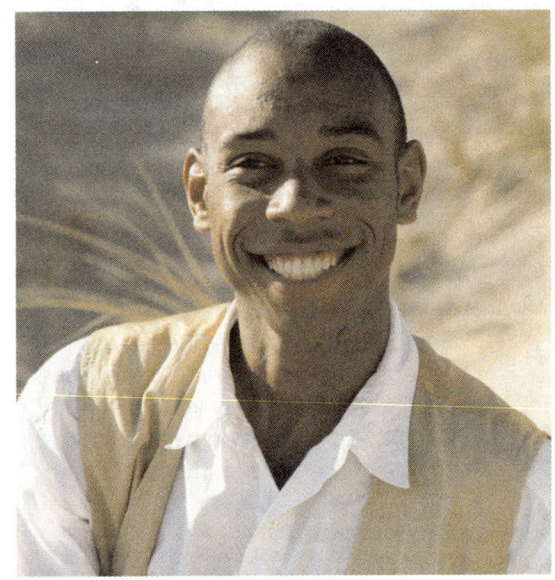

5-4 Before choosing to parent, a man should be sure he is mature enough to be an effective parent for his child.

A woman's age may also affect her readiness to parent. A young woman may feel she isn't prepared to handle the tasks of parenting. She might want to postpone parenting until she is more mature. This would give her a chance to meet more of her life goals. Another young woman might feel she is ready and mature enough to be a parent.

A man's age isn't really a concern in terms of the health of the baby. His age and maturity level do matter, though. Is he ready to be a father? Can he give the time and energy needed to be an effective parent? Is he mature enough to take responsibility for his child? See Figure 5-4.

Stability of Relationship

How secure is the relationship between you and your partner? Is it likely to last a lifetime? Children need a stable home environment. This is true whether they live with one or two parents. If parents have an unstable relationship, this affects their children. Some couples choose not to parent for this reason. Others choose to parent, but not to stay together as a couple.

Work or Career Factors

What work or career goals do you have? How would becoming a parent affect these goals? Would your desired career fit well with parenting? Jobs with long hours, travel requirements, or dangerous job duties often don't combine well with parenting. If this is the case for you, would you be willing to choose other, better suited work?

Finances

Raising a child is expensive. It takes money to pay for the food, clothing, health care, and shelter he needs. Your child will have educational and entertainment expenses, too. Can you and the baby's father support a child financially? Does at least one of you have a job that will provide for him? If not, how will you pay these expenses?

Feelings About Children and Parenting

Do you like children? If you're not a person who really likes being with children, parenting may not be the job for you. However, if you enjoy children and truly want to be a parent, this will make a big difference.

Ability to Provide for a Child's Needs

How able are you to meet a child's emotional, physical, intellectual, and social needs? Do you have a clear understanding of what these needs are? Are you capable of fulfilling your role as a parent? If not, you might wish to reconsider becoming a parent at this time.

Caring for a child is a big job. As a parent, do you have the support you'll need to help you meet these needs? An African proverb says "It takes a village to raise a child." This saying reflects the role of extended family, school, religious groups, and communities in meeting children's needs. Do you have enough support?

Ability to Provide Unconditional Love

Some people choose to parent because they are ready to give unconditional love to a child. Unconditional love is love for someone no matter what might happen. It means you will love your child just because she exists. No matter how she behaves, your feeling and expressions of love will not change.

Conditional love puts limits on when a person will love. For instance, a parent may express love only when the child acts as the parent wants him to act. The child may not feel loved unless she is doing what the parent wants her to do. Children deserve to have their parents love them all the time with no limits. See Figure 5-5.

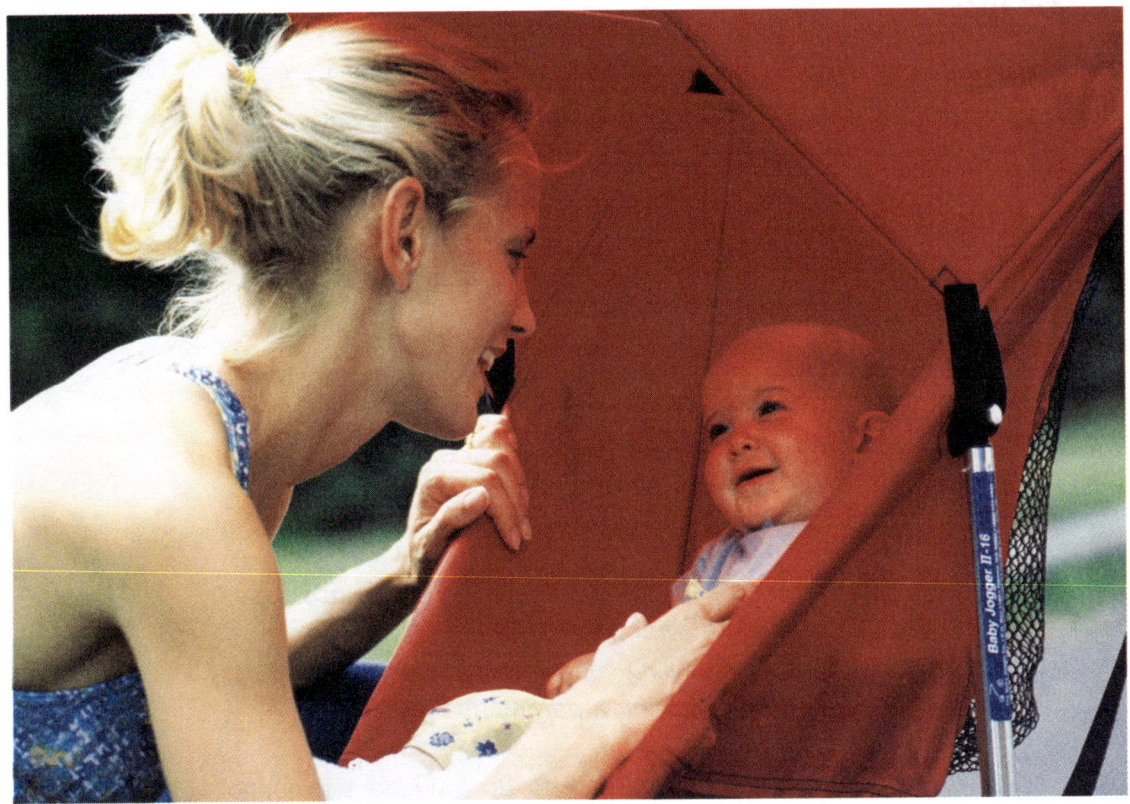

5-5 Showing unconditional love for your child can help her grow to be a happy and emotionally healthy person.

Am I Ready to Be a Parent?

When deciding about parenting, this is the question you really must answer. It can be hard to tell if you're ready to become a parent. Ultimately, you are the only person who can know for sure. It may take some time and a lot of thought to answer this question.

Many people don't think about whether they're ready to be parents. They just let it happen. Thinking things through is a sign of maturity, however. As you prepare to make your decision, ask yourself the questions on the following page.

- ☛ Do I really want to be a parent for the next 18 years? Do I want to take care of another person 24 hours a day, everyday? Do I enjoy being with children of all ages, from babies to teens?

- ☛ Am I ready for all the responsibilities of being a parent? Do I understand a child's physical, emotional, social, and intellectual needs at all ages? Am I prepared to meet these needs?

- ☛ Am I willing to make the sacrifices that parenthood may require? Am I willing to accept the limits it will place on my freedom? Have I done all the things I wanted to do before I begin parenting? Have I achieved my goals for my teen years? Am I willing to postpone or delay goals I had set for my twenties?

- ☛ What would I expect from my child? Will she be able to fulfill these expectations? What will my child expect from me? Can I fulfill these expectations?

- ☛ Am I able to be a sensitive, responsible, caring, loving, and understanding parent? Can I learn these traits if I don't have them? Which do I need to learn first?

- ☛ Is my relationship with my partner stable? Will it stand the strain of a third person who will consume large amounts of time? Have we talked about how a baby will change our relationship? Can we create a happy environment for her?

- ☛ Can I provide financially for a child? Am I prepared to offer a home, clothing, food, and supplies a child will require? If I have to work and go to school, how much time can I devote to my child?

Think about your answers to these questions. Do they reveal a readiness for parenting or the need to wait? If you choose to parent, do so because you want to be a parent and are ready for it. Don't just allow parenting to happen to you. Teens who don't think things through are the ones most likely to regret their decisions later. Take your time and make a wise choice. You will be more likely to be satisfied with this decision in the future.

Parenting Options for Teens

If you choose to parent, you have several options about how you will do this. You might choose to marry and raise your child with your spouse. Even if you don't marry, you might parent with your baby's father. Your family may be able to provide a lot of help whether you're married or single. Finally, you may choose to parent on your own. Each situation is unique. You, your baby's other parent, and your families can decide which option is right for you.

Within a Marriage

You and your partner may choose to marry and raise your child together. One big benefit of this option is your child would live in a home with two parents. This would likely be a stable home environment for him.

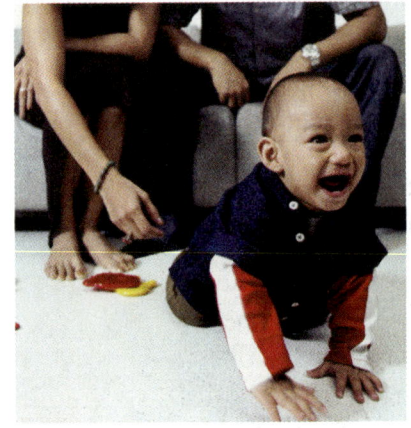

5-6 Being able to share the responsibilities and the joys of parenthood is an advantage of parenting within a marriage.

A second benefit is that married teens are partners. They will be sharing their lives together. This can make each parent feel more supported. It can also relieve some of the stress of teen parenting. Both partners can work together as a couple to make decisions for their family. They share both the responsibility and the joy of raising a child. See Figure 5-6.

Often, this option works quite well unless the marriage starts to fail. Constant fighting can take a toll on all the family members. The most negative effects are on the child. A child can sense when his parents are unhappy. This causes him stress, too.

Many married teen couples live with one partner's family. This arrangement can work well for young families, but it takes time and patience to adjust to it. The benefits of living with family may well outweigh the drawbacks.

Other married teen couples live on their own. This option is much more expensive, but it does have benefits. Teen parents may feel they have more authority over their children when they live on their own. Sometimes, though, they may feel isolated from the help their families can provide. Couples should choose the living arrangement that best fits their needs.

As Co-Parents

Suppose you and your child's father don't want to marry, but each of you wants to parent your child. This is common among teen parents today. It is called co-parenting. You and your child's father would not live together or share a romantic relationship. Instead, you would focus on being a parenting team for your child. Each of you would be a co-parent.

Even if the two of you aren't dating or married, both of you can still have your child's best interest at heart. You can work together to parent her and make decisions about her future. See Figure 5-7. One of you might be the residential parent, or the parent with whom the child lives. Her father could still spend time with her on a regular basis. In some cases, a child might live with each parent for part of the time. Each situation is unique, and co-parents have to figure out what will be best for them and their child.

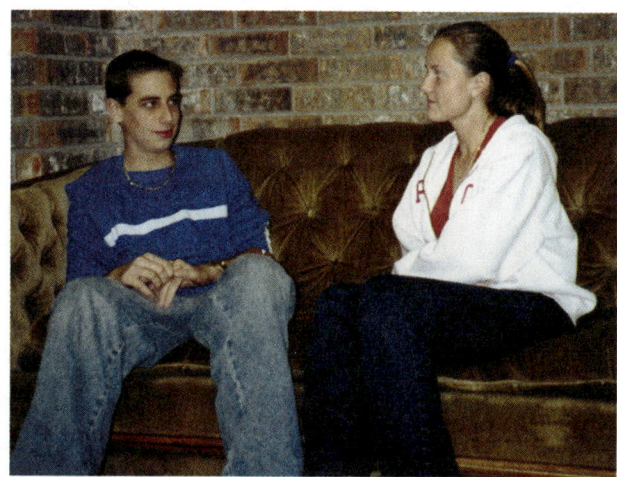

5-7 As co-parents, you and your baby's other parent can talk through major decisions affecting your child.

Co-parents might want to adjust their work schedules so they can share child care responsibilities. This gives both parents time with the child and reduces their child care costs. It can also ensure their child is receiving good care at all times.

Like marriage, co-parenting has the advantage of having both parents involved in the child's life. These two parents share the responsibilities and joys of parenting. They work together to raise their child. She can still be close to both of her parents and their families. Both parents give her the financial and emotional support she needs.

Often, this option works best when both co-parents are single. If either of them dates or marries someone else, it may cause hard feelings or complicate matters. If this occurs, it may take both parents and the child some time to adjust. Co-parenting is also difficult when the parents don't get along well. No matter how they feel about each other, co-parents need to work together for the sake of their child. If they have different views on raising children, this can cause problems. It can also be confusing for the child. Co-parents should talk about their differences and try to reach a compromise.

With the Support of Family

Many young parents rely on help from their own parents or other relatives. This kind of help is valuable for many reasons. First, you can learn from your parents' experiences in raising children. They can teach you quite a bit about parenting. Your parents spent many years guiding and raising you. They may remember what worked well and what didn't. Their advice may be helpful.

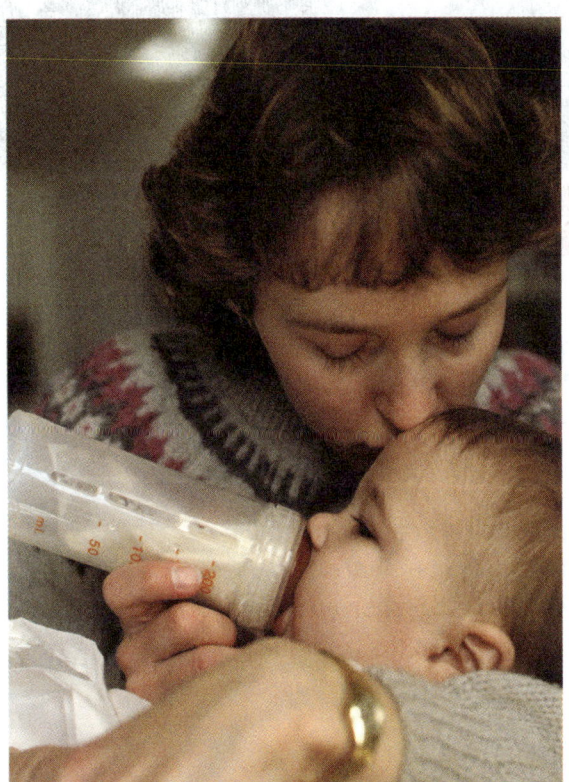

5-8 Knowing your mom is caring for your child can ease your mind when you must be away.

Second, you may not be able to afford to live on your own. Living with your parents can lift a great financial burden from your shoulders. It can allow you to use your money to meet your baby's other needs.

Third, your parents may be willing to assume some of the child care tasks that would normally be yours. They might help you with some daily care tasks or provide child care from time to time. If your parents are able, they might even care for your child full-time while you're at school or work. It would be comforting to know he's in good hands when you must be away. See Figure 5-8.

Parents and other relatives can also be a source of emotional support. You may be able to turn to them for advice and encouragement. They can listen to your concerns and share your joys. In times of need, your parents and other relatives may be willing to help.

Despite these benefits, there are also some drawbacks. Your parents' comments may sometimes sound to you like a "know-it-all" attitude. You may resent their efforts to guide you, especially when you disagree with their opinion. This may create tension in the family.

In addition, you will have to follow your parents' rules in order to live in their home. Your parents don't stop having expectations of you just because you have a child. At times, they may feel you aren't doing your part. They may think you're taking advantage of them. Arguments may result. For instance, if you aren't working, your parents may resent financially supporting you and your child. They may also resent it if you often leave him with them so you can go out with friends. This may interfere with plans they had made. If you and your parents argue often in front of your child, this can have a negative effect on him.

Living in your parents' home may also be crowded. This is especially true if you have younger brothers and sisters who also live at home. You and your baby might have to share one room. If you already share your room with another family member, it will be even more crowded when the baby comes.

Before your baby is born, talk to your parents about what help, if any, they are willing to provide. Be open with them about your needs and expectations. Find out what they need and expect, too. If they are not able or willing to help much, you need to know this right away. If they can help, talking about what everyone expects can help things go more smoothly.

It may also be a good idea to talk with a teen parent you know who chose this parenting option. This person can help you identify the good and bad points of the situation. His or her advice may help you see things more clearly. It may give you an idea of what to expect.

On Your Own

You also have the option of parenting alone. This is known as *single parenting*. Single parents have full responsibility for their children. Single parenting is very difficult. It means you would have to do all the tasks typically shared by two parents.

Single parenting may mean you can't rely on anyone else when making the many difficult decisions as a parent. You will have to decide matters by yourself and take full responsibility for your choices. This can be stressful. At times, you may wish you had someone else to help you make these decisions.

Single parenting may also mean you are the only person who is supporting you and your child financially. You must also supply the emotional, intellectual, physical, social, and moral guidance she needs. Single parenting is a big job.

There are advantages, however. For instance, you can raise your child as you wish without anyone else's input. Sometimes this is easier than reaching a compromise with your child's father. This is especially true if the two of you have different values and beliefs. See Figure 5-9.

Some single parents can afford to rent or buy a home. These single parents live alone with their children. This is an expensive option, but it does give the young family more space. Other single parents live with friends. Sometimes it works out well for two single parents to share a home as roommates. This can allow them to split their living expenses and offer emotional support to each other. As you decide where to live,

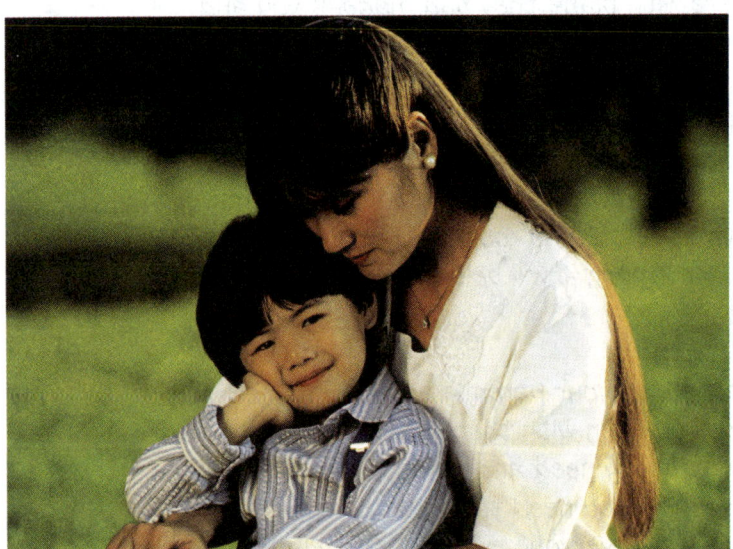

5-9 Being a single parent means you can make all the decisions regarding your child's upbringing. This is difficult, but it can also be an advantage.

consider your child's needs and your own needs. What are you able to do and what do you want to do? Choose the option you believe will work best for you.

Whether you live on your own or with someone else, you will have bills to pay. Maintaining a home costs money. You and your child will also have many expenses. Children need clothes, health care, school supplies, recreation, toys, and many other things. How will you meet these needs?

Will you work to earn money? If so, what training do you have or would you need? Can you earn enough to support your family? Who will care for your child while you are at work? How will you pay for this care? Do you have transportation to and from work and child care?

Can you rely on your family for any help? Will you seek aid from the state or federal government? Will you look to social agencies or your house of worship? Again, think about your child and what is in her best interest.

As a single parent, you will have to make many decisions on your own. If the child's father is involved, you may be able to consult with him occasionally. If you're close to your parents, you may want to ask them for advice and assistance sometimes. This kind of help will make your job as a single parent a little easier.

Even if you will be a single parent, your child's father has certain rights and responsibilities when it comes to your child. By law, both parents are required to financially support a child until she's an adult. With unmarried parents, paternity, or the biological fatherhood of a child, must be established. The father can decide to sign papers stating he is the child's father. If he won't sign these papers, he can be taken to court to prove paternity through DNA testing. Once paternity is established, the father receives parenting rights such as visitation. He is also then ordered to pay money to support the child. (To learn more about paternity, visitation, child support, and custody, refer to another title in this series, Building Your Future.)

Single parenting can be very rewarding, too. You and your child are likely to develop a very close relationship. As you watch her learn the things you've been teaching, you will feel rewarded. Watching your child grow and mature is fun. Single parents must remind themselves of these pleasures when they feel the frustrations that come with this difficult job.

Major Points

☛ Parenting is more than a title; it's a big job. A person may become a parent in several ways. No matter how he or she becomes a parent, though, this person has a duty to work to meet the child's needs.

☛ Parenting brings many adult responsibilities. Until your child is an adult, you are responsible for taking care of him. This can be challenging, but it is also rewarding.

☛ People choose to be, or not to be, parents for many reasons. This is a personal decision; the reasons vary for each person. Understanding what parenting involves can help you make the right decision for you.

☛ You may or may not feel ready to become a parent at this time. You can use the questions provided in the chapter to help you decide.

☛ Teens who wish to parent have many options. They can parent their child within a marriage, as co-parents, with the support of family, or on their own. You, the baby's other parent, and your families will make this decision based on your situation.

☛ Happily married teens may provide a very stable environment in which to raise a child. Being life partners makes parenting easier for these teens because each has the support of the other.

☛ Co-parenting means both parents working together to raise a child even though they are not married to or dating each other. This is a parenting partnership. Both parents share the joys and challenges of parenting.

☛ For teen parents, the support of family can be very beneficial. Their parents might be able to provide financial, emotional, and practical help. Many teens also appreciate being able to live at home with their parents.

☛ Some teen parents raise their children alone. These single parents have more responsibilities. This is an especially hard role, but it has advantages, too.

Chapter 6
An Important Decision

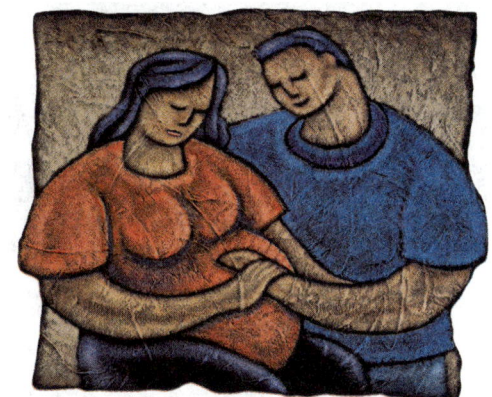

The early stages of pregnancy bring many choices. For teens, the biggest of these is whether to parent, plan an adoption, or have an abortion. This is a serious and permanent decision. It will change your life. You need to think carefully about what you will do. A well-made choice is rarely regretted in the years ahead. Hasty decisions may later lead to guilt, regret, and depression.

Talk to your partner and family about this decision. Their advice will matter to you. You may feel you need more help deciding what to do. If so, talk to a counselor, teacher, religious leader, or other trusted adult. They may be able to help you. The final choice, however, is yours to make.

You've already learned about parenting. In this chapter, you will learn more about your other options—adoption and abortion. This chapter will also guide you through making this important decision.

Parenting

One of your options is to become a parent. You may want to refer to Chapter 5 for information on what it means to be a parent. When you understand what parenting involves, you can decide whether this is the right choice for you.

If you become a parent, you will have a large responsibility. Your child will be depending on you. Almost everything in your life will change. If you're ready to accept both the good and bad aspects of being a parent, you can succeed in this role. See Figure 6-1.

After you choose parenting, you have many other questions to answer as well. Some involve other people. It would be wise to talk to them about these issues. These questions include the following:

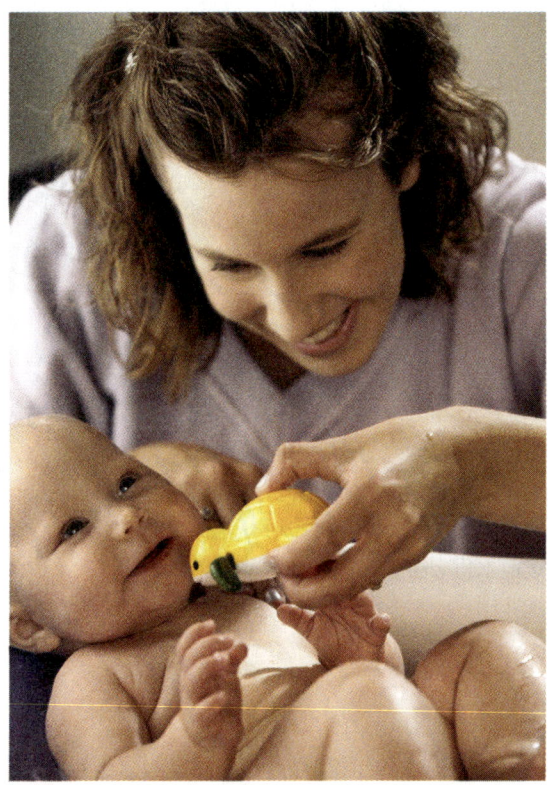

6-1 Teens can be good parents when they prepare for this role and have realistic expectations about what lies ahead.

- What will be the relationship between the baby's father and me? Will we marry, co-parent, or lead separate lives? Will he be involved with the pregnancy, labor, and delivery? Will he take the important role of father?
- What role will my family play? Will they be my primary support or will I do things on my own? Are they willing to provide any emotional, financial, or practical support? Can they help me with child care or parenting tasks?
- Where will the baby and I live? Will it be with the father, with my parents, with his parents, or on our own? If I must pay the rent or mortgage, how will I do this? If we will live with family, what can I do to make the adjustment easier?
- Will I be able to stay in school? Are there special classes, programs, or schools in my area for pregnant and parenting teens? Would these be beneficial to me or would I prefer to stay in my regular school?
- If I stay in school, who will take care of my child? Will I have to find a child care provider? If so, how will I pay for this?
- Will I work part-time to help pay my baby's expenses? If so, who will care for my child and how much will it cost? Will I make enough money to justify working?
- What community and government resources might be available to help me in my parenting role?

You will face these questions and more if you choose to become a parent. Once your baby is born, you face even more decisions about his care. At times, it may be difficult to sort out all these issues and make these tough choices. With patience and practice, you can make the best decisions for you and your child. Trust in your ability to be an effective parent. It won't be easy, but you can do it.

If you will be parenting, it's a good idea to learn more about your community resources. What local agencies can help pregnant and parenting teens? Do you qualify for public aid programs? If so, what help can these programs provide? Are there support groups or other parenting organizations you can join? When you have the help and support you need, you will feel less stress. You can concentrate on what's really important to you—parenting your child.

Adoption

In an adoption, birthparents transfer their role as parents to other adults, called the adoptive parents. The adoptive parents accept all legal rights and responsibilities for the child. They become his parents and raise him as their own.

An adoption can help all those involved. It gives the adoptive parents a chance to share their lives with a child. Being parents can enrich their lives. Adoption can help birthparents find a better life for their children than they think they could provide. At the same time, it allows them to fulfill their own life goals. The child will benefit, too. He will grow up in a loving home with parents who are ready and able to meet his needs. See Figure 6-2.

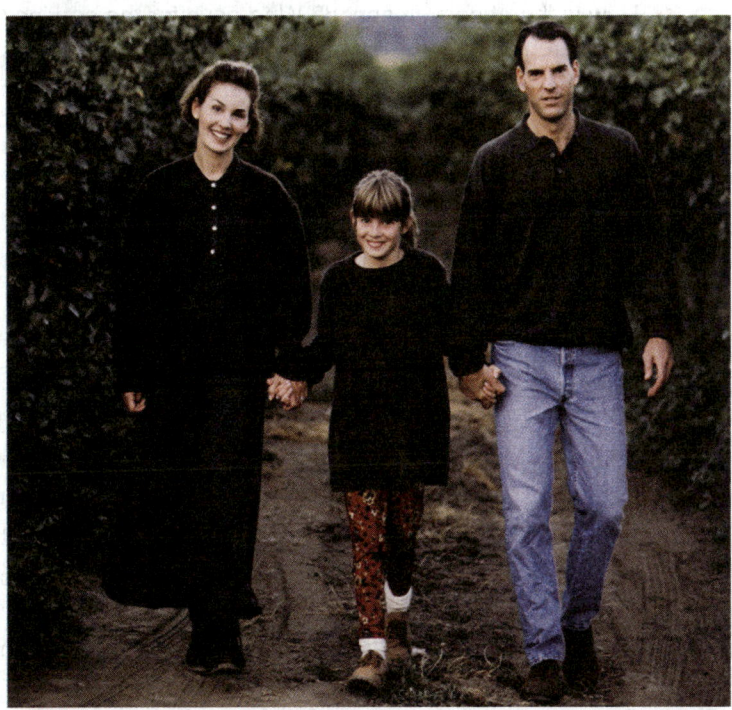

6-2 Adoptive parents are ready for the responsibilities of parenting. They can offer outings and special trips as well as meeting a child's basic needs.

Adoption is legal in every state. Each state sets its own adoption laws, though. You can contact the Child Welfare Information Gateway to learn about your state's adoption laws. This is a national agency that provides adoption information for the public. You can request information about adoption laws in your state. The more you know, the more informed your choice will be.

Adoption Agencies

An adoption agency is one that has been licensed by the state to help people plan adoptions. Two main kinds of agencies are public and private. A public adoption agency is run by the state government. This agency places children who are in the custody of the state. These children have been left or surrendered by their parents.

Checking out Adoption Agencies

Ask the following questions about each adoption agency you are considering:

- How is the agency financed? Who pays for the services provided? What charges must birthparents pay? What fees do adopting parents pay?
- What services does the agency offer the birthmother and birthfather before and after delivery?
- What services does the agency offer adopting families?
- How are adoptive families chosen?
- What role do birthparents play in selecting the adoptive parents?
- Does the agency arrange open adoptions? How are they carried out? Does the agency discuss the pros and cons of an open adoption?
- What types of problems and successes has the agency had with adoptions and placements over the years?
- What follow-up services does the agency provide for birthparents and adopting families throughout the adoption process?
- Does the agency provide each set of parents with copies of the materials given to the other?
- After delivery, what happens if the birthparents choose to parent their child?
- What type of counseling does the agency offer to help birthparents make the right decision for them regarding pregnancy?
- What care arrangements does the agency provide for the baby between the birth and the signing of the consent form (legal adoption papers)?
- Do you trust and feel comfortable with the people at the adoption agency?

6-3 Ask questions such as these when you visit adoption agencies.

Chapter 6   An Important Decision   109

Private adoption agencies are run by private groups instead of the government. Many are run by religious or nonprofit service groups. Others operate for a profit. State laws govern private adoption agencies. Each agency also has rules and policies of its own.

If you're thinking about adoption, find out what agencies are in your area. Visit each agency to see which is the best match. Choose an agency that makes you feel welcome and at ease. You want an agency where you will feel comfortable. The questions in Figure 6-3 can also help you choose an agency.

The next step is to talk with an adoption counselor at the agency. This person is trained to help you work through choices about your pregnancy. The counselor shouldn't tell you what to do. Instead, he or she will help you think matters through and choose the option you feel is right. Seeing an adoption counselor doesn't mean you agree to an adoption. It simply means you want to learn more and talk with someone who can help you decide.

Your adoption counselor can also help you find other help you will need. See Figure 6-4. Some agencies provide housing for pregnant teens. Most will pay your prenatal health care bills. This can help you have a healthy baby.

You can help plan your child's adoption. How involved you can be depends on the agency. Some agencies will ask what kind of parents you want for your child. You might prefer a couple of a certain religion or culture. The agency will choose an adoptive couple that meets your wishes. Other agencies will give you profiles of adoptive parents and let you choose. Ask what policies the agency has about this.

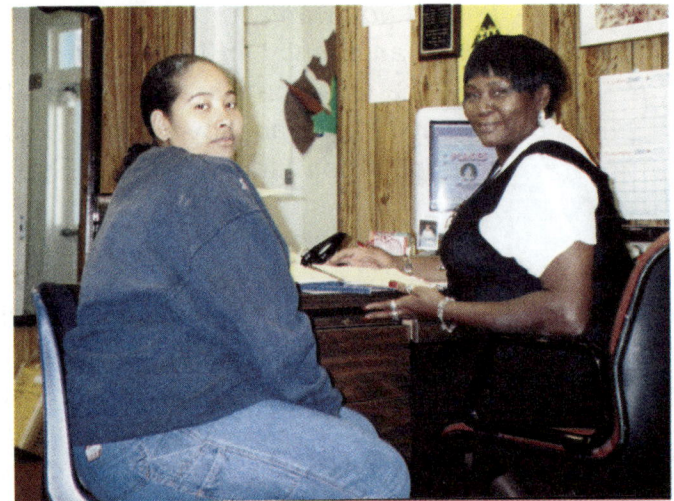

6-4 An adoption counselor can guide you through the process and help you find other resources you need.

You want the best for your baby. You may worry an adoptive home won't be safe for your child. Rest assured; agencies carefully screen people who want to adopt. They check to make sure the couple can provide a good home for a child. The agency will do a criminal background check on people wishing to adopt. They also contact many of the couple's references. The agency also does more than one interview with the couple. They ask about the couple's reasons for adopting and why they feel they can be good parents. The agency also asks about the parents' ages, income, and health.

Finally, the agency does a home study, or a visit to the couple's home. This visit ensures the couple has an adequate and safe home for a child. The agency looks at the condition and safety of the home. They check to be sure the home has plenty of space for a child. If the couple passes this study, they will become adoptive parents. Ask if your agency will let you see the home study report of the parents chosen for your child. Some agencies allow this. This might reassure you.

With so much screening, you can feel sure your child would be placed in a safe and loving home. If you still have doubts, talk to your counselor. Ask about the agency's screening process. This may ease your fears.

If you want to plan an adoption, it's a good idea to work with an agency. In this type of adoption, the agency will handle all the legal matters. You won't have to take care of these yourself. The agency will guide you through the process and support you along the way. This can be a big help.

Independent Adoption

Independent adoptions are ones that are not arranged through state-licensed adoption agencies. Many of these adoptions occur between family members. For instance, a stepparent may adopt the children of his or her spouse. In this case, the help an agency can provide isn't needed. The birthparents, adoptive parent, and their lawyers can take the legal steps needed to arrange the adoption. This type of adoption is legal in most, but not all, states.

An independent adoption can also be done through a doctor, religious leader, or lawyer. These professionals work with the public. They often meet couples who wish to adopt and birthparents who wish to plan an adoption. A doctor might match birthparents with a couple who wants to adopt. In this type of adoption, both sets of parents and their lawyers must handle the legal matters. They have more to do than if they had chosen an agency adoption.

Birthparents can also work with an independent adoption service. This is an organization that works with adoption, but is not licensed by the state. Be cautious when seeking an independent adoption service. The government does not regulate these organizations as much as it regulates adoption agencies. The quality of the help offered can vary quite a bit. Often, less screening of potential adoptive parents is done. This can be a concern for birthparents. Before using one of these services, carefully check into its reputation and business practices. Ask many questions about the kinds of help the service provides.

This type of adoption does have some good points. First, birthparents can often choose their child's adoptive parents. In some agency adoptions, they can't. Also, both sets of parents have more control in planning the adoption. As long as they follow state laws, they can set the terms they want. In agency adoptions, both sets of parents must follow guidelines and rules set by the agency.

Despite these good points, many professionals don't advise this type of adoption for teen birthparents. Independent adoptions often do not provide the support teens may need. Handling all the legal matters can be stressful. Teens need the help and guidance that an agency can provide.

A second drawback to this option is the lack of counseling. Often, this is not a part of independent adoptions. If either set of parents wants counseling, they must arrange it (and often pay for it) themselves. Many experts advise both sets of parents to seek counseling throughout the adoption process. Birthparents may need help working through their feelings about this choice. Adoptive parents may need help adjusting to the ways in which the adoption will change their lives.

Openness in Adoption

You also need to think about openness when making an adoption plan. *Openness* means how much contact you would have with the adoptive family. An adoption with no contact is a *closed adoption*. In this adoption, the two sets of parents have never met. They don't know each other's identity.

A closed adoption gives privacy to both sets of parents. Some people prefer this kind of privacy. They may not want to stay in contact or share any personal information. If so, they should choose an agency that will respect their wishes.

Until the 1970s, almost all adoptions were closed. Then, attitudes slowly started to change. Open adoptions became more common. In an *open adoption*, there is some kind of contact between the birthparents and adoptive family. How much contact varies greatly, though. It depends on the policies of the adoption agency.

The amount of openness also depends on the wishes of each set of parents. In most open adoptions, birthparents choose the adoptive parents. Both sets of parents may meet before the adoption. See Figure 6-5. They may choose the baby's name together. The birthparents might either invite the adoptive parents to be present for the baby's birth or let them visit the baby in the hospital.

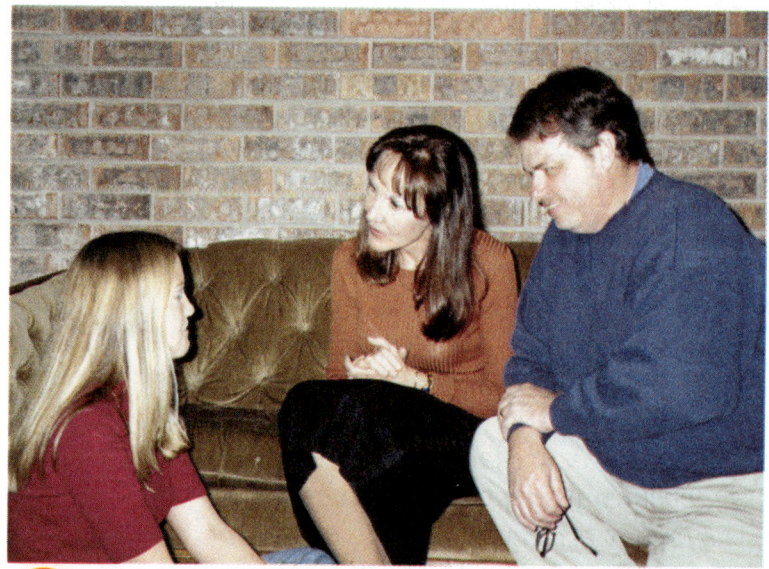

6-5 Some pregnant teens want the chance to get to know the people who will adopt their babies.

Chapter 6   An Important Decision

After the baby is born, both sets of parents may keep in contact through the agency. They can exchange letters and pictures. This still allows them to keep their last names, addresses, and telephone numbers private.

In some cases, both sets of parents keep in very close contact. They may see each other from time to time. Both sets of parents may spend special times together, such as the child's birthday or holidays. This allows the birthparents to see the child and be part of her life.

Some birthparents find this type of close contact difficult. It stirs their feelings about the adoption and doesn't let them find a sense of closure and peace. Others are comforted by this contact. They feel happy about the role they can play in their child's life. Watching their child grow up in a loving home reassures them they made the right choice.

When planning an adoption, you should decide how much openness you want. This is a personal decision with no right or wrong answer. Make your wishes known to your adoption counselor. Ask for adoptive parents who want this same amount of openness. Choose an agency that will let you have as much openness as you want. If you make an agreement with the adoptive parents about openness, keep your word. This is best for all parties involved with the adoption.

Reasons for Choosing Adoption

Teen birthparents may choose adoption for many reasons. Most often, they did not plan for the pregnancy to happen. They may not want, or feel ready, to be parents. Adoption can allow them to keep pursuing their life goals. Delaying parenthood may help them be better parents when the time is right.

Some pregnant teens and their partners see adoption as the only acceptable choice. These teens do not feel ready for parenting. They may not believe abortion is an option. Instead, they choose to give birth and place their child in a loving home.

Birthparents may also choose adoption because they can't financially support a child. They don't want their parents to have this burden. Teens may feel it's unfair to ask their parents to pay the costs of their pregnancy and support their child.

Teens most often choose adoption out of concern for their child's well-being. For various reasons, they may feel unable to provide what a child needs. Through adoption, they can give their child more than they feel they can offer. Considering their child's needs first is an unselfish choice.

The Adoption Process

In both types of adoption, the same legal steps occur. After the baby is born, you and the birthfather would sign some papers. These papers would allow the adoption agency or adoptive parents to take the baby from the hospital. Next, paperwork must be filed with the court. These papers state that both sets of parents want the adoption to take place. On these forms, you and the birthfather will sign your consent to the adoption. The baby is then placed with the adoptive parents. In most states, you cannot change your mind after giving your consent. Other states allow you to change your mind within a short time after the signing of these papers. You'll need to check the laws in your state.

The last step is the final adoption hearing. At this court hearing, the judge declares the adoption final and legal. The court orders the baby's original birth certificate to be sealed. A new one is made that lists the adoptive parents as the baby's parents. When the child is an adult, he might be able to get a copy of the original birth certificate listing his birthparents. Again, laws vary among states.

Your adoption agency can tell you more about this process. You can also see another book in this series, Building Your Future, to learn more about the legal aspects of adoption.

Feelings About Adoption

If you plan an adoption for your child, you may have mixed feelings. Denial, anger, guilt, and deep sorrow are common in the first few months after an adoption. You will likely grieve for a time.

Chapter 6 An Important Decision   115

This is normal, even if you feel you're doing what is right. You may miss your child and wonder how he is doing. In time, this pain will lessen. This may be of little comfort at the time, though. See Figure 6-6.

You may also feel some peace and a sense of relief. The long adoption process has ended. Your child is in a loving home where his new parents will take very good care of him. Feeling good about this can help. If you didn't expect to feel this way, it might also make you feel a little guilty.

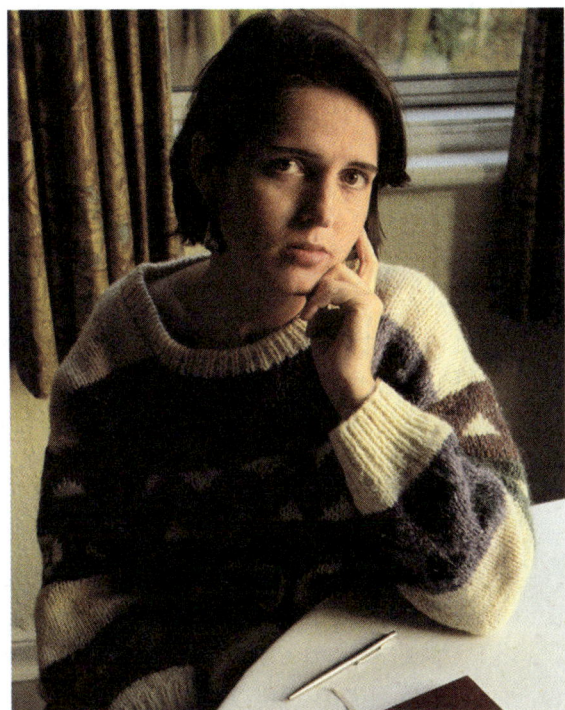

6-6 Planning an adoption is an emotional decision. You may feel more sad than happy for a while, even if you feel you're making the right choice.

Most adoption agencies provide support groups to help birthparents cope with these feelings. Attending a support group for teen birthparents can be comforting. You know each of these teens has made an adoption plan and may share some of your feelings. A support group can give you someone to talk to who understands what you've been through.

Counseling can also help you manage your feelings about the adoption. Your adoption counselor has helped other teen birthparents through this process. This person is familiar with the kinds of feelings you might have and how you might cope with them. He or she can listen and help you sort out your feelings.

If you choose adoption, you may feel pressure from others to change your plans. Friends and family members may not understand why you're choosing this. They may accuse you of being selfish and not loving your child. Support groups and counselors can help you learn how to respond to these statements.

Your family and your partner's family may also have very strong feelings after the adoption. Family members may feel the loss, too. This child would have been a member of their family. Their grief may not be as intense, but it is just as real. Counseling may help them deal with these feelings. Try to be understanding about what they may feel.

Abortion

Some teens choose to end their pregnancies by abortion. Abortion is the removal of an embryo or fetus from the uterus to end a pregnancy. This medical procedure should be done in a hospital or clinic by a trained professional. Any other type of abortion is illegal. This includes trying various ways to end your pregnancy yourself.

A teen might choose an abortion for several reasons. She may have health problems that could be made worse by pregnancy and delivery. A woman may choose abortion if she learns her baby would have a severe disability. She may end a pregnancy that was the result of rape or incest. Finally, a woman might choose an abortion because she doesn't want to continue her pregnancy.

Abortions are legal in every state. The laws about them vary from state to state, though. Some states allow abortions throughout pregnancy. Most restrict them after the first three months. In some states, a waiting period is required from the time a woman applies for an abortion until the time she is allowed to have one. This gives her extra time to be sure of her choice. In other states, before a teen can have an abortion, her parents must be notified. If you're thinking about abortion, find out what the laws are in your state. (For more information on the legal aspects of abortion, see another title in this series, Building Your Future.)

The topic of abortion is very controversial. Most people have strong opinions on this issue. Many people do not believe it is right. Others support a woman's right to choose. Both sides agree that abortion should not be used as a form of birth control. For a woman's physical and emotional health, it is better to prevent a pregnancy than to end one.

Chapter 6   An Important Decision

Medical Issues

Abortion is a medical procedure. Before choosing this option, a woman should learn what is involved. Her doctor should explain everything to her. She should understand exactly what will happen and what the risks are. It's important to ask questions about anything that is unclear.

The most common method used to perform an abortion is vacuum aspiration. It can be used in the first three months of pregnancy. In a *vacuum aspiration*, the doctor causes the woman's cervix to dilate. A suction tube is then inserted. This tube is rotated around the walls of the uterus to remove its contents. The procedure takes about 30 minutes. The woman can return home the same day.

Most early, legal abortions are medically safe. There is a slight risk of complications, though. Be sure to think about these risks when deciding about abortion. With vacuum aspirations, the most serious risk is *sterility*, or the loss of the ability to have a child biologically. This could result if the uterus or cervix is damaged in the abortion. This risk is rare but serious.

The risk of other possible complications is pretty low, too. See Figure 6-7 for a list of other risks. Some of these are minor and don't last long. A woman should contact her health care provider, however, if she has any of these symptoms. This will ensure she gets the medical care she needs.

Medical Complications of an Abortion

Several medical complications may occur after a vacuum aspiration abortion. These include the following:

- excessive bleeding
- cramping
- fever or infection
- chills
- muscle aches
- tiredness
- abdominal pain
- backache

6-7   If you choose an abortion, these are the medical risks you would take.

A second option to cause abortion is mifepristone. This medicine blocks a hormone that sustains the pregnancy. It must be prescribed by a health care provider in the first seven weeks of pregnancy. The woman takes mifepristone once in the provider's office. She must return to the provider two days later to take a second medicine that will cause the uterus to contract. The combined effects of these two drugs should end the pregnancy. At a third visit about two weeks later, the provider tests to find out if the pregnancy has ended. If it has not, further options are discussed at this time. This method ends pregnancy in 92 to 95 percent of cases.

When mifepristone is used, cramping and bleeding are the most common side effects. Bleeding often lasts 9 to 16 days, and should lighten each day. In a few cases, surgery may be required to stop very heavy bleeding.

Emotional and Social Issues

Deciding whether to end a pregnancy isn't easy. This decision is serious and permanent. It deserves a great deal of thought. Take your time. Be sure you've made the right choice for you.

Many emotional and social issues tie into abortion. You should think about these when deciding whether this is the option for you. The sections that follow describe a few of these issues.

Personal Beliefs

What are your personal beliefs about abortion? Do you feel it's an acceptable option? Pay close attention to your feelings. This is an area where your choice should match your values. Otherwise, you won't be comfortable with this decision later. It might cause you grief or guilt in the future.

You may feel you need help clarifying your personal beliefs. If so, you might want to talk to a counselor. This person can help you sort out how you feel. Talking to your religious leader may help you understand faith issues related to abortion. This, too, may help you decide.

Your Reasons

What reasons do you have for considering an abortion? Be clear with yourself about why you might choose this option. This will help you make the best decision. Given your reasons, do you think abortion is the best option?

Partner's Wishes

What does your partner think about your pregnancy and the option of abortion? He may be pushing you to end your pregnancy. If so, be sure you don't choose abortion only to satisfy him. Be sure it's what you want, too. On the other hand, your partner may want the two of you to parent the child. If you are still together, his opinion will matter to you. See Figure 6-8. It can affect your relationship if he doesn't agree with the choice you've made. In the end it's your decision, though.

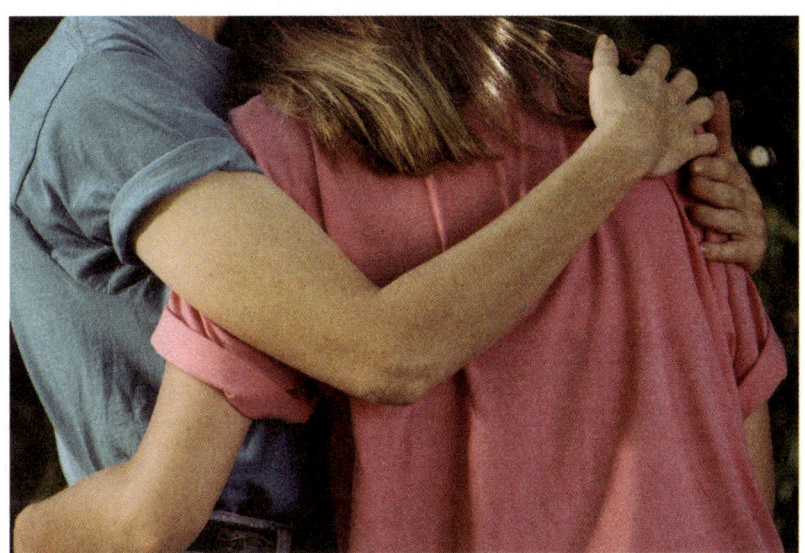

6-8 If you and your partner are still together, having his support is important.

Support of Important People in Your Life

Your partner's opinion isn't the only one that will matter to you. Other important people in your life will have strong feelings about this, too. If family members and friends disagree with your choice, it may cause problems in your relationships with them. It is good to think about this beforehand.

If you're thinking about abortion, you will probably want to discuss it with your parents. This can be difficult, but you'll want to know where they stand. This is especially true if you live in a state where their permission is required.

Future Effects

How will choosing an abortion change your life? Is this a decision you can live with a year, 5 years, or 10 years from now? Do you think you will suffer lasting grief and regret? Will you be comfortable with this choice and grateful for the chance to keep pursuing your life goals? Are you willing to take the medical risks?

Thinking Through the Decision

As you think about your future, you know a big decision lies ahead. This choice will change your life. It is a serious and permanent decision. Take your time and consider your options very carefully. You want to make the best decision you can regarding your pregnancy.

At first, you may wonder how you can ever make such a huge decision. One way is to use the decision-making process. (You may want to refer to Chapter 3 to review this process.) Making important choices can be tough when your emotions are involved. The decision-making process is a logical approach that can guide you through making the right choice for you. The following six steps make up the decision-making process.

Identify the Decision to Be Made

In this first step, you commit to deciding what you will do regarding your pregnancy. You have decided you're ready to resolve this issue. This step shows your willingness to consider your options and reach the best decision for you.

Gather and Examine Information

In this step, you're learning all you can about the decision you face. Talk with other people who have experienced teen pregnancy. Listen to authorities, such as teachers, counselors, and doctors. Find out what the important people in your life think about the issue. Do some research. Go online or check out books and magazines from your school or public library. See Figure 6-9. Write all this information on paper so you can organize it and refer to it later. The more information you have, the better decision you can make.

Identify Your Options

Now that you know more, you can identify what options are available to you. For this choice, your main options are parenting, adoption, or abortion. (Each option has many other choices within it. Here we are only considering which main option you will choose.)

Evaluate Each Option

In this step, you will consider each option for its potential to work for you. List the advantages and disadvantages of each option. Share your lists with two or three adults you respect. Ask these adults what other advantages and disadvantages you may not have considered.

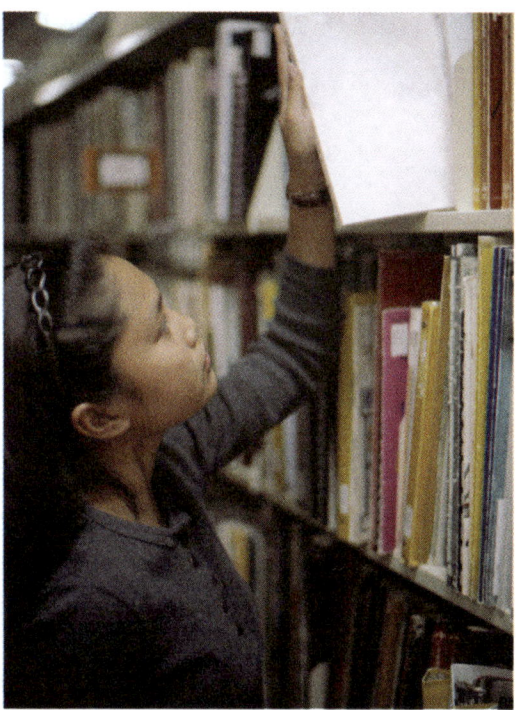

6-9 You can research to learn more about the decision you face. Being well informed lowers your chances of making a decision you will regret later.

What are the consequences of each option? Are you willing to accept these? For instance, what do important people in your life think about the decision? You don't have to base your choice on other people's opinions, but you do need to think about how this decision will change your life. It may affect your relationships with others. Not having the support of those close to you can be difficult. If you choose an option they don't support, you will have to accept this.

Next, think about your values and goals related to this decision. How does being pregnant relate to your values? Which options support your values and which conflict with them?

What goals do you have for your life? How would each option affect these goals? Whichever option you choose, you should be willing to accept the effects it will have on your goals and values.

The last part of this step is to eliminate any options that won't work for you. These are options that have consequences you're not willing to bear. Also get rid of options that will affect your goals and values in ways you cannot accept. These are not good choices for you.

Choose the Best Option and Act on It

Select the choice you believe is best. Develop an action plan. What steps do you need to take? Which will you do first? A written action plan may be the easiest to follow. This way you can check off each item as you do it. It also makes it easy to see what your next step will be. See Figure 6-10 for an example of a written action plan.

After you've formed an action plan, it's time to put your choice in motion. Begin working on the steps you've identified. Follow through with the choice you've made.

Evaluate the Results of Your Decision

In this final step, you need to review your decision. This might occur some time after the decision is made. Did you choose the right option? Would you make this same choice again in the same circumstances? What would you do differently? What can you learn from this experience?

Action Plan: Adoption

- *Choose an adoption agency and make an appointment with an adoption counselor.*
- *Talk with Terry about decision to plan adoption.*
- *Talk with Mom and Dad about decision to plan an adoption.*
- *Make a list of the characteristics I want in the family who raises my baby.*
- *Decide on the level of openness I prefer.*

6-10 An action plan like this one can help you carry out the decision you've made.

Chapter 6   An Important Decision

Accept responsibility for your decision. Do not blame anyone else. This can be hard, especially if others pressured you to make a decision they felt was right for you. You own the decision, however. The mature thing to do is to take responsibility for it.

Deciding what to do regarding your pregnancy may be one of the hardest choices you'll ever make. If you take your time and think matters through, you can do it. Following the decision-making process can guide you to the decision that's right for you.

Major Points

- Many decisions lie ahead for you. The biggest is what you will do regarding your pregnancy. You can choose to parent, plan an adoption, or have an abortion. This is a serious decision that will change your life. Take the time to make it carefully.

- If you choose parenting, you will take on an enormous amount of responsibility. If you're ready and committed to being a good parent, you may find much joy in this role as well.

- If you choose adoption, you will transfer your rights and responsibilities as a parent to adoptive parents. This can give your child what you may not be able to provide right now.

- Working with an adoption agency is a wise choice for teen birthparents. An agency can give you the support you need and guide you through the adoption process. Having someone handle the legal matters for you is a benefit of this option, too.

- Independent adoption is an option for birthparents in most states. It is not often recommended for teen birthparents, however. The lack of support, counseling, and guidance can make this a more difficult option for the birthparents.

- Openness refers to how much contact occurs between the birthparents and the adoptive family. Some adoptions are closed, with no contact occurring. In an open adoption, some type of contact occurs. How much contact varies from one adoption to another.

- The adoption process is a series of legal steps that occur to make an adoption final. Laws governing this process vary from state to state. Often, it includes completing many forms, as well as having a final adoption hearing.

- ☛ You might have mixed feelings about planning an adoption for your child. It's not easy, but these strong feelings will lessen in time. Counseling and support groups may help you through this difficult time.

- ☛ If you choose an abortion, you will need to make this choice relatively early. Many states restrict abortions after the first trimester. You might also need your parents' permission. Be sure you know what will happen and what risks are involved. Think carefully about the possible emotional and social effects of this decision.

- ☛ The decision-making process can help you choose what to do regarding your pregnancy. Take your time, and carefully consider all the options and the consequences they bring. You will want to talk to important people in your life about this decision, but in the end the choice is yours. Make the decision you feel is right for you.

Part Two
Your Changing Relationships

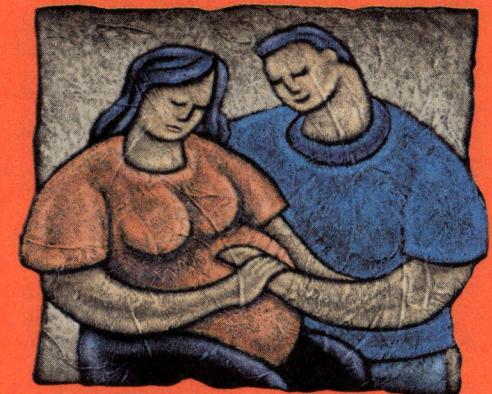

One small person brings many big changes! At first, there is much excitement. Soon, you'll discover how becoming a parent seems to disrupt everything. All areas of your life require some adjustments, including your relationships with others. Even though these relationships change, they're still important. You can do much to strengthen your relationships with others. The final four chapters of this book will serve as a relationship road map by

♣ describing adjustments you can expect in early parenthood,

♣ helping you evaluate your relationships,

♣ emphasizing responsible sexual decision making,

♣ encouraging you to examine your communication skills, and

♣ informing you about crises that can sometimes occur in relationships.

Chapter 7
Adjusting to Life as a Teen Parent

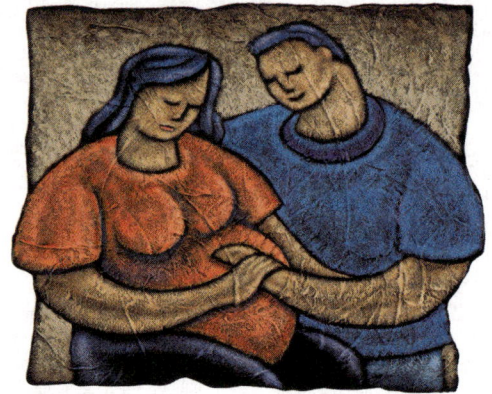

Becoming a parent means making some changes in your lifestyle. You will need to adjust many aspects of your life to meet your baby's needs. As your life changes, so will your relationships. This can cause the expectations you have for others to change. It can also cause them to change their expectations of you. All these adjustments and changes can bring stress into your life. This chapter will help you learn about how your life will change and how you can deal with stress.

Comparing the Roles of Teen and Parent

You are both a teen and a parent. Sometimes these roles may conflict. As a teen, you want to do the fun things your peers do. On the other hand, you also want to be the best parent you can be. It may seem like these two desires clash. Is there a balance, a happy medium? Can you fulfill your roles as a teen and a parent? Will you be able to meet your baby's needs and still fit in with your friends?

Think about what it means to be a teen. What do you expect from your teen years? See Figure 7-1 for a list of expectations most teens have. Simply put, you probably expect to spend your teen years preparing for adulthood. Getting your high school diploma, holding a job, and forming relationships help you prepare to be an adult. These tasks require you to focus on yourself and your development as a person.

Chapter 7 Adjusting to Life as a Teen Parent

The pattern for most teens is to live at home with their parents. As they gain maturity, their parents allow them more responsibility and freedom. At some point, they are ready to go out on their own and "try their wings."

Now look at your expectations of being a parent. Refer to Figure 7-1 again for a list of common parenting expectations. As a parent, your task is to provide care and guidance for your child as she grows. You want to help her become a healthy person. In parenting, the focus should be on your child and how you can help meet her needs.

Unlike the gradual process of a teen becoming an adult, parenthood is immediate. Once you're a parent, you have all the responsibility at once. You may feel unprepared to accept it all right away. It is okay to accept help from others. If you live with your parents, family members, or your partner, they may be able to help you adjust to this new role.

Comparing the Roles of Teen and Parent

Expectations as a Teen	Expectations as a Parent
completing high school and perhaps continuing your education; participating in school activities and events	providing for your child's basic needs (clothing, shelter, food, safety, and health care)
dating, having friends, having fun, and taking time for yourself	giving daily care to your child (feeding, bathing, dressing, comforting, and supervision)
being a family member	guiding your child toward healthy physical, intellectual, emotional, and social development
having a part-time job	helping your child grow to meet her full potential
learning adult tasks such as driving, working, and caretaking	being the head of your family (you and your child)
working to reach physical, intellectual, emotional, and social maturity	handling adult tasks, such as driving, working, and caretaking

7-1 Becoming a teen parent means you have competing roles to fill.

Are any of the parenting expectations the same as those of being a teen? No. That is why these roles sometimes conflict. You may want to do one thing, but know you need to do another. For example, at one time you may consider these three options—spending time with your baby, studying, or going out with your partner or friends. Which is most important? All three are important but you must choose. Many people believe that, for parents, time with their children must come first.

Adjustments a Baby Demands

When your baby is born, your lifestyle must change a great deal. Your baby is totally dependent on you. He is helpless and can do nothing for himself. You must feed, bathe, and dress him. He even needs you to change his position so he can get comfortable. Your baby needs you to do everything for him. See Figure 7-2.

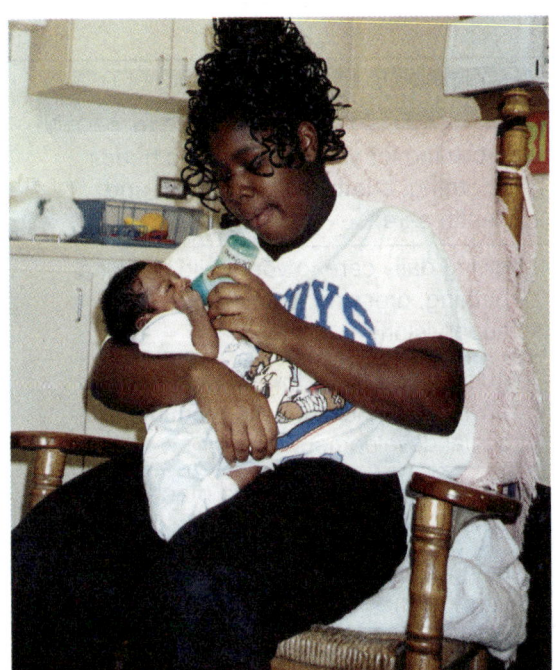

7-2 Feeding your baby several times each day is only one of the many ways being a parent will change your life.

As a teen, you're probably used to taking care of yourself first. You may have never been totally responsible for the care of someone else. Perhaps you've helped take care of younger brothers and sisters, but your parents probably still had most of the responsibility. Suddenly, you must put your child's needs ahead of your own. This may seem unnatural at first, but with practice it will be easier.

This is one of the biggest adjustments you will have to make as a parent. Because you're still growing and developing, too, this is a delicate balance. You'll need to develop management skills to help you make the most of your limited time and money. This will also help you juggle school, work, and child care responsibilities.

Chapter 7   Adjusting to Life as a Teen Parent

Managing Your Time

When you become a parent, your use of time must change. Your baby depends on you to meet her needs. This means changing your schedule. Some of the time you used to spend on your own interests must now be devoted to caring for your baby.

For the first several months, your baby may get hungry often at night. If so, someone must get up to feed and diaper her. This can mean giving up your own sleep, which can make you tired. Adjusting to this new routine can take some time. It may affect how much you feel you can get done during the day. Concentrating at school or work on a few hours' sleep can be difficult.

Then, when you come home from school or work, your baby needs to be fed, bathed, dressed, and cuddled. Her clothes and bottles will have to be washed. The diaper bag needs to be packed and ready for the next day. See Figure 7-3.

Diaper Bag

A diaper bag for a newborn should include everything you'll need to care for the baby until you return home again. You may not need all the items listed here, depending on your baby and the situation. However, most diaper bags for newborns include all or most of the following:

- 4 to 6 diapers (short outing) **OR** 8 to 12 diapers (all-day outing)
- wet wipes or wet washcloth in a resealable plastic sandwich bag
- diaper rash ointment
- changing pad
- adequate number of prepared bottles (include 1 to 2 extra) **OR** 1 to 2 prepared bottles and enough extra formula to make the rest
- 1 to 2 toys to entertain the baby
- 1 to 2 clean cloths or burp rags
- 1 to 2 changes of clothes
- 1 to 2 clean undershirts
- 1 to 2 plastic bags for dirty diapers or clothes
- 1 to 3 pacifiers, if your baby uses them
- beloved object (blanket, stuffed toy), if your baby needs it
- medicine, small receiving blanket, hat, jacket, and bib, as needed

7-3   What should you pack in your newborn's diaper bag? This can depend somewhat on your child's needs, the weather, and the size of the bag.

Now it's time to start on homework. This routine is demanding. You may wonder how to find time for yourself, family, dating, and friends.

How can you make time to do everything you need to do? You must prioritize, or decide which things are most important. To help you do this, write a list of all the tasks you want to do in a day. Beside each task, write the amount of time you think you'd need to complete it. Add up the amounts. Do they equal more than the 24 hours you are given each day? They probably did, which means you are trying to do too much. This activity demonstrates you can't do everything. Too much is asked of you in the amount of time you have. This is why you must set priorities. It helps you focus your time and energy on the tasks that matter most to you. Be sure your priorities match your long-term goals for you and your child.

Once you have established your priorities, you can set a basic schedule. This schedule will include time each day or week for those things that matter most to you. See Figure 7-4. Set aside time for your baby and the care she requires. Include time for school, work, and homework. Pencil in a block of time for yourself. Keep adding important items to your schedule until it is fairly full. Don't forget to leave a little time completely free each week. You can use this time to do whatever else needs to be done.

A schedule will serve you and your baby well. First, a schedule takes away the guesswork of what to do next. You won't worry as much about how to find time for everything. Your schedule represents your best solution to this problem. This can reduce your level of stress. Your child will also do best when her world is predictable. She will feel safest when she knows what is coming next. Having a routine will also help her know when it's time to relax and fall asleep. This will make bedtime easier for both of you.

Use your schedule as a guide, but be flexible. It is okay to stray from your schedule sometimes. A special event or an emergency can cause your schedule to change. If you live with your family or your partner, you may sometimes need to adjust your schedule to meet their needs. If this special need passes, you can go back to

Kim's Example: Managing Time

Kim is a teen mom. She cares for her baby, goes to school, and has a part-time job. Kim was feeling overwhelmed by all that was expected of her. She made this chart to see where her time was going. After completing the chart, it was clear to Kim she was doing all she could and the other things that were expected of her would have to wait until the weekends when she had more free time.

1 a.m.	2 a.m.	3 a.m.	4 a.m.	5 a.m.	6 a.m.
Sleep	Sleep	Sleep	Feed baby Go back to sleep	Sleep	Wake up, shower, and dress
7 a.m.	**8 a.m.**	**9 a.m.**	**10 a.m.**	**11 a.m.**	**Noon**
Feed baby and eat breakfast Pack diaper bag and backpack Take baby to child care	Take school bus to school **8:30** School starts	School	School	School	School (Lunch)
1 p.m.	**2 p.m.**	**3 p.m.**	**4 p.m.**	**5 p.m.**	**6 p.m.**
School	School	School **3:30** Pick up baby from child care; go home	Play with baby; relax	Feed baby and eat dinner **5:45** Go to work (baby stays with grandma)	Work
7 p.m.	**8 p.m.**	**9 p.m.**	**10 p.m.**	**11 p.m.**	**Midnight**
Work	Work	Go home Bathe and dress baby Put baby to bed	Do homework	Do homework	Go to sleep

7-4 Use Kim's schedule as a guide to set your own. This will help you manage your time your regular schedule. If it doesn't, you can adjust your regular schedule to include it. Following a schedule most of the time will help you manage your time well.

Managing Your Money

Learning to manage your money wisely is the key to success. This will take some practice if it is new to you. Before you were a parent, you may have been able to spend your money for whatever you wanted. Your parents might not have placed many rules on how your money was to be used. Now, however, you have many more demands on your limited finances. You must find a way to make your money meet your needs and your child's needs.

Using your money wisely requires self-control. This is the ability to monitor your own actions and make appropriate choices. An example of showing self-control is not buying new clothes for yourself because you know your child will soon outgrow his clothes and need more.

Thinking of another person's needs first may be new to you. Having to account for where all your money goes may be new, too. You may have never had to keep up with how your money was spent before. Taking on financial responsibility for your child can be difficult. Your baby needs to have his basic needs met. Food, clothing, shelter, and health care are essential. As a parent, it's your responsibility to make sure these needs are met.

If you don't have enough money to meet your child's needs, visit your local public aid office. You might qualify for some financial help. Even if you don't like the thought of being on aid, it can be a valuable resource for you and your child. Meeting your child's needs should be a higher priority than avoiding embarrassment or clinging to your pride rather than seeking help. Your partner and family may also be able to help you with money.

To make the most of the money you have, you'll need to set up a budget, or spending plan. This budget will help you plan how to pay your bills and buy the things you need. Keeping your budget in mind will help you keep from overspending. When you manage your resources poorly, it can lead to many problems. It means you will not end up having enough money to buy all the things you and your baby need. Both of you would have to go without some things. It is not fair to deprive your child of what he needs because you spent money foolishly. In serious cases, this is considered child abuse and neglect. By learning to manage your money wisely, you can avoid these and other money-related problems. (See another title in this series, Building Your Future, to learn more about money management.)

Managing Your Schoolwork

Schoolwork is often a challenge for teen parents. In order to get it completed, you must make it a priority. When friends are calling or there's a good ballgame, it may be hard to focus on homework. Concentrating may be even more difficult when your baby is crying or needs your attention.

Even the things that used to be simple are now more complicated. Getting ready in the morning now includes feeding and dressing your child. When you pack your backpack, you may have to pack a diaper bag, too. If your child is cared for outside the home, you'll have to take her there. This extra trip may mean extra time and hassle at the start of your day. If your child can receive child care at your school, this means hauling your backpack, baby, and diaper bag to school. This can make getting on and off the bus a struggle. Be sure to allow yourself extra time to arrive early.

Schoolwork will also be harder to keep up with now that you're a parent. You have so many demands on your time, and they all seem important. Think of your education as your ticket to a future career that can support you and your child. This will help you keep things in perspective. Your schoolwork deserves the most attention you can give it.

You can take steps to make managing your schoolwork easier. The first is to use a planner, small calendar, or notebook to keep track of your assignments. See Figure 7-5. Some schools give planners to each student. If your school doesn't provide one, you can buy one or create your own. Any small book or calendar with plenty of space for writing will work. Take this with you to all your classes. Simply write the assignment on the date it is due. You can also block off time to do the work. Setting goals and time for doing your assignments will help you feel more in control of your life. If you find a goal can't be met, try to adjust your schedule and fit it in at another time.

Good school habits include setting a time each day to do homework and review what happened in class. For many students, the best time is shortly after arriving home from school. After a brief

Using a Calendar to Manage Schoolwork

Sunday	Monday	Tuesday	Wednesday	Thursday	Friday	Saturday
		1 Science- do review questions	**2** Science- review questions due; study for test	**3** Math-p.43 due Science- study for test	**4** Science- Test!	**5**
6	**7** English- Choose term paper topic	**8**	**9**	**10** English- Start library research for paper	**11**	**12**
13 English- Research	**14** English- Research	**15** English- Research	**16** History- Study for test English- Research	**17** History- Study for test	**18** History- Test!	**19**
20	**21** English- Write rough draft	**22** English- Rough Draft	**23**	**24** Math- Study for test English- Start revising rough draft	**25**	**26** English- Finish final draft
27 Math- Study for test	**28** Math- Study for test	**29** Math- Test! English- Print paper	**30** English- Paper Due!	**31**		

7-5 Note how this student uses a calendar to write in assignment due dates and block out time to do the work.

break, snack, or time with the baby, these students sit down and review the day. They organize the tasks to be done by the next day and plan for any long-range assignments. Some students tackle the hardest work first in order to get it over. Others start with the easiest work in order to feel successful. You may want to try both methods and decide which works best for you.

If you can, set aside a space at home to do your homework. Choose a quiet place where you can spread out your books and papers and leave them undisturbed. This can be a good way to get more work done if you only have short time blocks. For instance, you might be able to fit in a few minutes of homework while your baby naps and a few more when she plays nearby. Sometimes these short bits of time can really add up.

If your home isn't comfortable for studying, you may need to find another quiet place. Your public library may be a good option. While you're at the library, you need to stay focused, though. When your work is done, perhaps you can reward yourself by going online, reading a magazine, choosing a book you'd like to read, or just relaxing for a few minutes.

At times, it may be impossible to finish an assignment when it is due. Your child may take up all the time you had planned to study or an emergency might arise. At times like these, it's important to set priorities. Most teachers will be more understanding if you do part of your homework than none at all. You may get points taken away for what you didn't finish, but in many cases, this is better than nothing. Learning the skills the homework covers also matters. You might choose to skip the part that is easiest for you. Spending time practicing or studying the hardest part may be a better use of time. Many teachers will appreciate your effort if you explain why you made this choice. Your teacher probably knows your situation and admires you for doing the best you can. If not, you can still take pride in knowing you did your best and acted responsibly by talking to the teacher about it.

Keeping a Part-Time Job

Many teens have part-time jobs to help them pay for some of the things they want. Often teen parents must work to help meet the needs of their children. Teens who attend school and also work may feel stressed and tired. This is even more true for teen parents, who have the responsibility of caring for a young child.

It is wise to set limits on how many hours you will work per week. Working too many hours can lead to high levels of stress. It can deplete the energy you need for school and parenting. This can cause you to fall behind in class or neglect your child's needs. Setting limits helps you keep everything in perspective.

Your state may have a limit on the maximum number of hours you can work while enrolled in school. This is a starting point. The limits that are right for you might be even lower than this number, though. This is because you have the added responsibility of a child. When you accept a job, make your supervisor aware of your limits. If your employer can't respect these limits, you'll need to find a different job.

You may need to use your planner or calendar to help you keep track of your work hours. This will help you remember which days and what hours you're scheduled to work. It can help you see conflicts with your other obligations. You can see at a glance when you might have to hire a babysitter or ask for a day off work.

If you want to keep your job, you'll need to develop positive work behaviors. You'll want to show your supervisor you're dependable and reliable. This type of employee uses the behaviors shown in Figure 7-6.

Qualities of a Good Employee

- arrives at work on time
- comes prepared and focused
- dresses appropriately for the job and is well-groomed
- keeps his or her word and follows through
- displays a positive attitude
- gets along well with boss, coworkers, and customers
- does the job as well as he or she can
- follows directions and accepts constructive criticism
- adheres to the policies of the employer
- takes breaks of proper times at appropriate times
- admits to mistakes and avoids blaming others
- cleans up work area before leaving
- works until the assigned quitting time
- notifies the boss as soon as possible of any needs for time off

7-6 Which of these qualities do you have? Which should you work more to develop?

Are you this kind of worker? If you are, you will become a valued employee. Your supervisor will respect and appreciate you. (See another title in this series, Building Your Future, to learn more about finding a job and succeeding in the workplace.)

Finding a Good Babysitter

When you're at school or work, your child will be with a child care provider. This person will take care of him on a regular basis for an extended period of time. Your parents or a friend may provide this kind of care. Most often, it is given by a child care center or family child care home. (See another title in this series, Helping Your Child Grow and Develop, to learn more about child care.)

Once in a while, you will need a babysitter. This is a person you will arrange to have care for your child for a few hours or days at a time. Babysitting is short-term care. You may need a few hours to focus on a school project. You might want someone to watch your child so you can go to a school function or social event. A sitter can also take over for a day or two if your child care provider is unavailable.

Many teen parents are fortunate. They have friends or family members who will babysit once in a while for free. Parents take turns babysitting each other's children. For instance, it might work for a neighbor to watch your baby one week and you to watch her child the next. You could trade babysitting for the same number of hours. This is a way parents can keep costs down. At times, however, you may have to pay someone to stay with your child.

How can you choose a good babysitter? It is good to have a person with some training and experience in caring for young children. An organization such as Girl Scouts, 4-H, or the American Red Cross may run a training class for babysitters in your community. Hiring someone who has had this class may reassure you. Another option is to hire a classmate who is in an early childhood or child care class. A third idea might be a neighbor or friend you know who works as a babysitter. You can also check with other parents for recommendations.

Before you hire a babysitter, you may want to see this person interact with your child. You might invite him or her to come over and play with your child while you're home. This lets you see how the babysitter and your child get along. It can help you decide whether you'd feel safe leaving your child with this person.

You can also ask a prospective babysitter for references from local people for whom they have worked. You might also ask what he or she likes about children and finds hardest about caring for them. These questions will give you insight into what to expect. If you feel satisfied with the person you have chosen, you can ask him or her to babysit for you. Be sure you go over important information with your babysitter before you leave your child in this person's care. See Figure 7-7.

Changing Expectations in Your Relationships

In a relationship, you expect the other person to act and respond in a certain way. Some of this is based on what you want from the relationship. What you know about the other person also plays a role. This person has expectations of you, too.

What Your Babysitter Needs to Know

- Where you will be, when you expect to return, and how to contact you (tell the sitter whether to answer the phone or door and what to tell callers or visitors regarding your absence)

- Instructions regarding meals, snacks, bedtime, medical needs, rules, restrictions, and guidance techniques (instruct the sitter which foods, drinks, and other items are okay for him or her to use such as the phone, TV, stereo, computer)

- A tour of the house (including first aid supplies, safety devices, and possible escape routes)

- A list of emergency phone numbers (including those of nearby relatives or neighbors) and a medical release form (allows the sitter to authorize medical care for your child in an emergency)

Keeping your babysitter informed can help things go smoothly for him or her and your child while you're away.

As a parent, you're taking on a new role. This causes changes that affect your relationships with others. What each of you expects from the other may change. At first, this can cause friction in the relationship. If you can talk openly to others about these changes, your relationships with them can adjust. This takes time, effort, and patience, though.

With Your Family

When a baby is born, every member of the family takes on new roles. This is an adjustment for the entire family, not just the new parent. When you became a parent, your parents became grandparents and your siblings became aunts and uncles. Adding these new roles can be confusing. What new expectations should accompany them? This is a difficult question, and each family answers it differently.

Think of several items lined up straight in a row. This straight line represents the family and each individual item is a member. If one person changes, (moves out of the row), it can upset all the others because their view of their family must change. The members have to adjust this view in order to still work together as a team. This can take time. Your family is the same way. As your life changes, your family members must change, too.

This is especially true when you live with your family. A new baby in the house may affect their daily routines and lifestyle. If your baby stays in your room with you, a sister who shares your room might have to give up some of her space for the baby. People might have to be quieter when you're trying to put the baby to sleep. Crying in the night may awaken everyone.

You and your parents might have talked before the baby came about each of your expectations for taking care of your child. If not, now would likely be a good time to do this. Tension will be lower when everyone is clear on how responsibilities in the house will be split.

Your parents will likely expect you to be responsible for both you and your child. They may not want to be involved much in her care. Your parents may tell you they have already raised their children and this one is all yours. They might expect you to do your child's laundry and keep her things picked up and neat.

On the other hand, your parents might expect to share much of the daily child care tasks with you. They may offer to care for the baby while you're in school or at work. Your mom might get up with her some nights so you can get more sleep. Your parents might expect to help guide and discipline your child as well.

Before your child was born, your parents probably expected you to behave like other teens. They saw you as just a regular teen who was preparing for adulthood. Now, however, they may see you differently. You have chosen to take on the adult responsibility of parenting. People often think of parents as always behaving in an adult way. For this reason, your parents may now expect you to act like an adult.

You're still a teen, though. You won't always act like an adult because you're not finished growing or developing. The concerns and emotions you have are still related to being a teen. You're still learning how to be an adult. At times you may be confused about how to behave. Your parents may be confused, too. They may resent it when you act like a teen because their expectations of you have increased.

Some other questions you will need to discuss with your parents include the following:

- ☞ Will the baby's father and his family be allowed to visit?
- ☞ Will you still be allowed to have friends over?
- ☞ How would your parents feel about you dating?

Until you talk with your parents, you won't know where they stand on these types of issues. Even if you're nervous, it's best to get these topics out in the open so you can discuss them. Afterward, everyone will likely feel some relief.

If your parents offer their help with parenting your child, this can be reassuring. Your parents have experience and can give you advice. See Figure 7-8. In fact, being asked for their advice and guidance can make them feel valued and needed. You can learn from your parents' successes and mistakes. On the other hand, you don't want your parents to tell you how to raise your child. If they're constantly telling you how to do things, you may resent this. In time, you and your parents will likely find balance in this area. Talk to your teacher or a counselor if the relationship between you and your parents is abusive or the communication is very poor. Perhaps this person can assist you in finding the help you need.

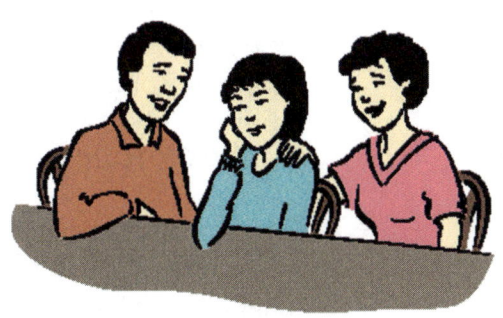

7-8 Talking to your parents can help you learn more about raising a child.

If your mother shows a willingness to help, be careful not to take advantage of her. Avoid making unreasonable requests for her, such as having her care for your baby every night so you can go out. This isn't good for you, your baby, or your mother. It doesn't help you mature or bond with your baby. It may confuse your baby about who is her parent, which can lead to jealousy between you and your mother. Your mother has already raised her children. She also needs time for herself and other members of the family.

Your brothers and sisters may also treat you differently after you become a parent. They may resent the extra attention you get. Your relationship with your child may make them jealous. Depending on their age and maturity, they may try to help you. Other times they may try to push you away. You will need to help them understand your new role as a parent. Also spend time strengthening your relationship with them. Remind them they're mportant to you and your baby.

Communication is one of the best ways to keep your family relationships strong. By sharing your concerns, feelings, and expectations, you can understand each other better. (See Chapter 3 to learn more about communication.)

Being patient and forgiving with family members will also help. Expect there to be many adjustments and even disagreements along the way. Try your best to see the other person's point of view and help resolve these problems. This will improve your relationships with your parents, siblings, and other members of your household. It will also set a good example for your child.

With Your Co-Parent

You and your baby's father will have expectations of each other as parents. This is true whether you marry, live together, date, or are uninvolved. What you expect depends on what your relationship is like. If you're still together, you may expect him to be very involved with you and your child. If you're not together, you may want him to co-parent, or share parenting with you. Perhaps you want him out of your lives completely. What you and your family expect from your baby's father influences the role he will play.

Much also depends on what role he is willing to play. Your child's father has expectations of you and of his role. He may expect you to take care of everything so he can be out of the picture. At the other extreme, he might want to parent the baby by himself. He might be willing to co-parent with you, marry, or live together.

It is important to discuss what your expectations are. Both of you need to be clear about how much financial, physical, and emotional support you can offer your child. You may have talked about this during your pregnancy. If not, now is the time to do so. Try to reach an understanding on how involved each of you will be in parenting your child. See Figure 7-9.

If you have a good relationship, it will be less difficult to have this talk. However, if you're not on good terms, you may need a third person to help you

Shirleen Joe and Jason Tsosie, GRADS program at Newcomb High School

7-9 It is important for you and your co-parent to discuss how you will share parenting responsibilities.

work things out. This person can keep you focused on the issues. He or she can also diffuse any anger you feel toward each other.

If you and your baby's father are co-parents, what roles will he play? The answer to this question will differ for each family. For the most part, he can play whatever roles the two of you agree upon. This is why it's good to discuss the expectations you each have.

In almost all cases, a teen father is expected to provide money to help support his child. This money pays for the housing, food, clothing, health care, education, child care, and other items for his child. The father has a legal responsibility to pay child support. Some teen fathers willingly accept this role. Others must be taken to court and ordered to pay.

If a father doesn't pay after being ordered to do so, he can be taken back to court again and again. Once a court order is made, the child support payments are due even if the father doesn't have a job or is in school. The process is lengthy, and it can be tough to get all the money owed even with a court order. There is no time limit on collecting this money, though. The father can be taken to court for it again in the future when he has a better-paying job. (For more information on child support and related issues, see another title in this series, <u>Building Your Future</u>.)

Beyond money, a teen father should also provide some of the daily care for his child. For instance, he might feed, bathe, dress, diaper, or soothe his infant. With an older child, he might cook, read stories, and play outside. He might help guide and discipline his child. If he doesn't live with the child, he can still offer this care when he and the child are together. He may want to introduce the child to his family and have the child visit with these relatives. Knowing both sides of the family can help the child feel even more loved.

If the father lives with the child all or part of the time, he'll give much more of this daily physical care. In some families, children divide their time between living with their mothers and with their fathers. How long they live with each parent differs. Fathers might have the children with them for as long as six months or as little as a few days at a time. Some children live with one parent during the school year and the other in the summer. In a few situations, fathers take total responsibility for their children. The children live with them all the time. This might happen when a mother can't, or doesn't want to, parent the child.

Another common role for teen fathers is providing love and emotional support for their children. Many teen fathers love their children and want to be there for them. They spend time holding, kissing, hugging, and being close to their little ones. A father's nurturing and attention is very good for children. It can stimulate their brains to grow and help them feel good about themselves.

Fathers are also role models for their children. (This is true whether they realize it or not.) Many children copy the actions and words their fathers use. They imitate their fathers because they love and admire them. Children, especially boys, may even want to be like their fathers.

Mature teen fathers take responsibility for their actions. They want to become good parents for the children they have fathered. These young men are willing to do what it takes to meet their children's needs. They will try to cooperate with their children's mothers as co-parents. These fathers offer their children all they can.

The best arrangement for a child is to have both a mother and father who are involved and care about him. This is true even if his parents don't live together or share a romantic relationship. For this reason, both parents should try to work together as a parenting team. Each of you has much to offer your child.

The two of you can try to share decisions about how you will guide and discipline your child. If you agree on these issues, it will be better for your child. He will know both of you have the same rules. If you talk about parenting issues, it can also help you understand each other better. Good communication skills are vital for co-parents.

Do what you can to encourage your baby's father to get involved. He may feel left out or unsure about how to help. This is true whether he lives with you or not. It will be more of a problem if he doesn't live with you, though.

You can do much to include your child's father in his life. First, be considerate and respectful of him. Work together to decide on times for the child to visit him. Unless you have a serious cause for concern, let him have some time with your child on his own. He might take the child out or to his home for visits. This can help him feel like they have a separate relationship. This can also make things go more smoothly if the two of you don't get along so well. See Figure 7-10 for more ideas on encouraging your child's father to participate.

Involving Dad

If you and your child's father do not live together, you may wonder how you can help him become more involved in your child's life. You're the best judge of what's appropriate for your situation, but some of the following tips might be useful:

- Promote the special relationship your child shares with Dad. Talk positively about your child's father in the child's presence. Allow the child to share happy thoughts and feelings about Dad with you.
- If possible, let Dad and his child talk on the phone for a few minutes each day. This gives their relationship a sense of connection and routine. If Dad lives far away, maybe you can encourage them to exchange letters or postcards.
- Encourage Dad to spend time with his child. Try not to make visitation an unpleasant event for Dad by starting an argument with him or being rude.
- Give Dad a written schedule of the child's day. This lets him know what goes on in the child's life. Encourage him to keep the same schedule when the child is with him. This consistency will help the child feel more at home with Dad.
- If the child attends child care, introduce Dad to the child care provider. This makes Dad feel involved in his child's care.
- Ask Dad's opinion when decisions must be made regarding your child. Let Dad help you make some of these decisions.
- When you take pictures of the child, have an extra set of prints made for Dad. This will make him feel valued. It may also bring him closer to the child.
- Create a journal or scrapbook of milestones in your child's life for Dad. This can help him feel more involved if he doesn't see the child every day.
- Allow Dad to introduce the child to his family members. Keep in communication with them, if possible, and encourage them to be involved in the child's life. When the child is older, help the child make artwork for relatives and write to or call them.
- Give Dad ideas of how he can help. He may not know how he is needed, even if he wants very much to help.

7-10 Dad is important in your child's life. Make the extra effort to include him when possible.

Involving him in these ways will make him feel more comfortable about being a father. He may be more willing to help with the baby when he knows what would be helpful. He will get to know your child better and understand his needs. By including your child's father, you help make him an important part of your child's life. Your efforts may help bring the two of them closer together. This can benefit each of you, especially your child.

With Your Partner

If you and your child's father are no longer together, you might be involved with someone else. You may have started seeing this person while you were pregnant or after your baby was born. Your relationship with him might not be that serious. He might be just someone you like to spend time with and go out with once in a while. On the other hand, he might be someone you're becoming quite serious about. Most relationships fall somewhere between these extremes.

Most likely, this is a relationship that matters to you. You probably gain support and enjoyment from your partner. It can make you feel good to have someone care about you, especially if your baby's father really didn't. As long as you keep balance in mind, having a partner relationship can be good for you.

It may be hard to make time for this new person in your life. Perhaps you can set aside one special time each week when you can see one another. Throughout the rest of the week, maybe you can see each other at school or talk on the phone. You have much to do, and you need to stay focused. Your schoolwork, job, and parenting tasks must come first.

Avoid the temptation to spend all your free time with your new partner. You will be excited about getting to know him and will want to spend lots of time with him. Even so, your baby won't need your attention any less because you're dating. Your other priorities shouldn't change, either. If you spend too much time with your partner, you may push away your friends and family members. These are the people who will be there for you even if your relationship ends. Be sure to take time to spend with them, too.

You will also want to avoid choosing an unhealthy relationship. This kind of relationship might make you happy in the beginning. Before long, though, it will only lead to unhappiness. Be sure you've chosen someone who cares about you as much as you care about him. Take things very slowly. It takes time to really get to know what a person is like. Use both your brain and your heart when making relationship choices.

You might wonder about bringing your child around your new partner. Your baby or young child might become very attached to your partner. If the relationship ends abruptly, this will be hard for her. For this reason, it is likely best to wait quite a while before introducing your partner to your child. Be fairly sure this relationship will last before you encourage a relationship between them.

With Your Friends

Social life is important to most teens. Before you were a parent, you probably spent a great deal of time with your friends. You might have gone with them to school dances and games, the movies, the mall, and out to eat. These activities were a fun way to spend your free time.

Now that you have a child, there is more to consider than having fun and doing what you want. You will also have much less free time than before. Caring for your baby takes up much of your evenings and weekends.

Keep in mind friendships change as people do. From the beginning of your pregnancy, your life has been in a constant state of change. Your friendships may have changed while you were pregnant. Some may have grown closer, while others probably faded away. The same will happen now that you're a parent.

You may find yourself feeling jealous of your friends. They don't have the same time constraints or responsibilities as you do. They can still be focused mainly on themselves. Your friends may also feel uncomfortable around you now. They may find it hard to relate to your concerns. At times, they may not know what to say to you. They may feel you are too focused on your baby and don't care as much about them anymore. All these factors may cause hard feelings between you and your friends.

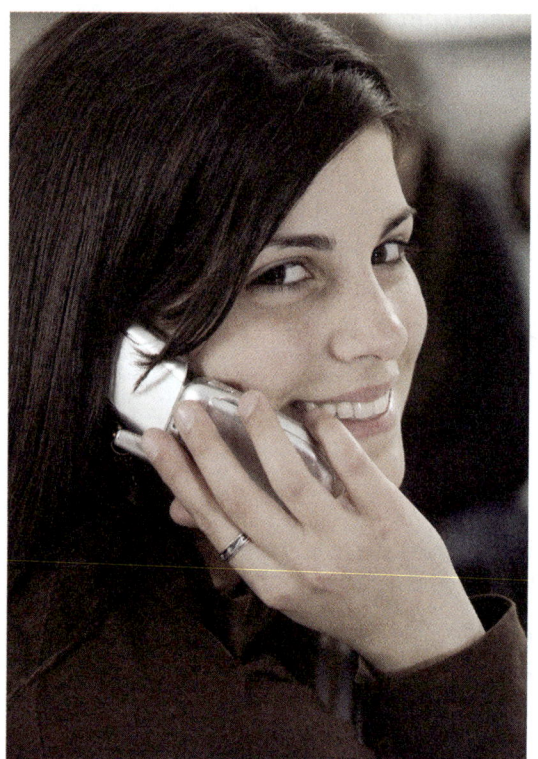

7-11 Talking on the phone can be a good way to spend time with friends.

Be sure to talk to your closest friends about how your relationship is changing. Tell them how much you value their friendship. Share how difficult it is to have quality time with them because of your new responsibilities. Ask them to suggest ways you can spend time together. Invite them to your home. Take your baby on walks with you and your friends. Spend what time you can together at school. You may be able to eat lunch, walk to classes, or sit on the bus together. Other times you may have to settle for just talking on the phone. See Figure 7-11. However you can, put in the effort it takes to stay close to them. Your true friends will be a support to you in good and bad times.

If you can find a babysitter, once in a while it will be nice to spend time with your friends without the baby. This will allow you to devote some attention to your friendships. It also helps you meet your personal needs of having some fun and relaxing. You can't expect a babysitter (or your parents) to watch your child all the time, though. It's also unfair to drag your baby with you to events that aren't appropriate for him. Your baby won't enjoy loud places, being outdoors in extreme temperatures or bad weather, or being out during naptimes or past bedtime.

For these reasons, you need to be choosy about which events you'll attend. You may also need more notice of activities so you can arrange for a sitter in advance. When you have a baby, you can't jump up and go places at the last minute.

Some close friends from your past will probably continue to be important to you. Making new friends is also a good idea. Try to make a few friends who are also young parents. They are the most likely to share many of your concerns. Friendships often develop when people who have common interests spend time together. It is easiest to meet other parents if you attend an alternative program or school for pregnant and parenting teens. You can also meet them in support groups through your community center or house of worship.

Dealing with Stress

All human beings face stress at times. Stress describes the tension you feel as a response to change. While you adjust to parenting, you may feel large amounts of stress at times. The changes you experience can stir up intense feelings.

Even positive changes can bring stress. This kind of stress may enhance your performance or drive you to do well. Think of the jittery feeling you might have before giving a speech. This type of stress is good for you because it encourages you to succeed.

Negative stress, or distress, is a more harmful kind of stress. It doesn't boost your performance. Instead, it gets in your way. This is the kind of stress described by the phrase stressed out. You will want to limit the effects of this type of stress. Knowing how to deal with stress can keep it from overwhelming you. Developing skills to help you manage stress is part of a healthy lifestyle.

Causes of Stress for Teen Parents

What causes stress to occur? No one answer applies to everyone. Stress is your body's reaction to change. You will respond to certain changes more easily than others. The changes that stress you out may not bother another person, and vice versa.

A stressor is a source of stress. One kind of stressor is a major life event. This is a happening that brings great change into your life. Pregnancy, childbirth, and becoming a parent are major life events that bring stress. Some of this stress is positive, while some can be negative. It can take some time to adjust to major life events and relieve the stress.

Daily hassles are a second kind of stressor. These are little annoyances and stresses you face from day to day. Traffic, transportation problems, waiting in line, and unfriendly sales help are examples of daily hassles. When these occur one at a time, it is easy to recover from them. When many occur at once or the same one occurs every day, this can cause your stress level to rise.

Many of the same stressors are common among teen parents as a group. You may be affected by many of these. In general, the stress teen parents feel centers around six main areas. These are school, relationships, time, money, work, and parenting concerns. See Figure 7-12 for examples of stressors in each area.

Common Stressors for Teen Parents

Parenting Concerns
- dealing with crying, fussing, poor eating, illness of baby
- lack of experience meeting a child's needs
- lack of sleep reduces energy to be given to parenting
- having to go to court to settle parenting matters
- dealing with your co-parent (if you're not together)
- finding an acceptable child care arrangement for your child
- adjusting to child care and being away from your child
- physical burden and rush of transporting a child and diaper bag to and from child care

School
- finding quiet time and place to do homework
- lack of sleep reduces energy to be given to schoolwork
- missing school if your child is sick or you don't have child care
- extracurricular activities
- keeping grades up

Work
- lack of sleep reduces energy to be given to job
- demands of supervisor or job
- long or late hours causes fatigue
- having to call in sick if your child is ill or you can't find child care

Relationships
- changing expectations between you and others
- disagreements with family, friends, co-parent, or partner
- lack of time to spend with friends or partner
- loss of the ability to relate to friends due to changes in your life

Money
- not having enough money to pay bills
- dealing with child support and public aid offices
- unexpected expenses
- having trouble balancing and sticking to your budget
- problems with creditors

Time
- feeling overwhelmed by all there is to do
- lack of time to relax
- changes in schedule
- unexpected demands on time

7-12 Which of these are stressors for you? What other stressors can you identify?

What are your stressors? What events or situations cause you the most stress? Some of these will be obvious to you. Over time, you will be able to recognize others.

Effects of Stress

In large amounts or over long periods, stress can affect your physical and emotional well-being. It can cause many problems that, in turn, can lead to even more stress. This can be a vicious cycle. By keeping your stress level low and trying to keep stress from lasting for long periods, you can minimize these effects.

Each person experiences stress in his or her own way. Some can handle much more stress than others. The effects of stress also vary from person to person. One may experience more serious effects than another.

The effects of stress fall into two groups—physical and emotional. Stress almost always causes some type of physical reaction. First, your body may experience the *fight or flight response*. This is the body's attempt to fight off the cause of stress or escape from it. When your body has this response, your heart and breathing rates will increase. Your blood pressure will rise, your muscles will tense, and you may begin to sweat. You may feel startled and overly sensitive to your surroundings.

You don't have any control over the fight or flight response. It occurs automatically when you are alarmed or under a sudden, unexpected stress. You might have this reaction right before a test or when you narrowly avoid a car accident. When you start to feel safe again, your body will calm down and return to its normal state.

Prolonged stress has different physical effects. The following areas can be affected by stress:

- Your <u>immune system</u> (the body system that fights disease) can weaken over time. This lowers your resistance to illness and infection. You might be more likely to get a cold or the flu when you're under stress.

- Your muscles may stay tense, especially in your jaw, upper back, and neck. This can lead to headaches and other discomfort.

- Your digestive system might be upset, causing a stomachache, nausea, or diarrhea. Eating habits may also be affected. You might eat less than you need if your stomach isn't feeling well. When you're stressed, food may not sound good to you. On the other hand, you might deal with stress by overeating or eating the wrong foods. Any of these responses can make you feel tired and sluggish.

- Your concentration may be impaired if thoughts of the stressor keep racing through your mind. This can affect your ability to focus on tasks as well as your sleeping patterns. You might either not sleep well or feel you need to sleep much more than normal. Changes in the amount and quality of your sleep affect your energy level and concentration.

Along with physical effects, stress can cause emotional effects. When you're under a lot of stress, you might feel unable to control your emotions. Instead, you might feel controlled by fear and anxiety. You might cry more easily or have a short temper. It's possible you might clam up and hide all your feelings. You might also feel frustrated and confused. Some people become depressed and hopeless when they've felt high amounts of stress for a long time. See Figure 7-13. They feel out of control and unable to see past right now. If you start to feel quite depressed, talk to a professional about these feelings. Maybe this person can help you resolve some of your stress.

What effects do you feel from stress? How do you know when your stress level is rising? Being aware of how you react to stress will help you recognize stress when it occurs. This is the first step to managing the stress you feel.

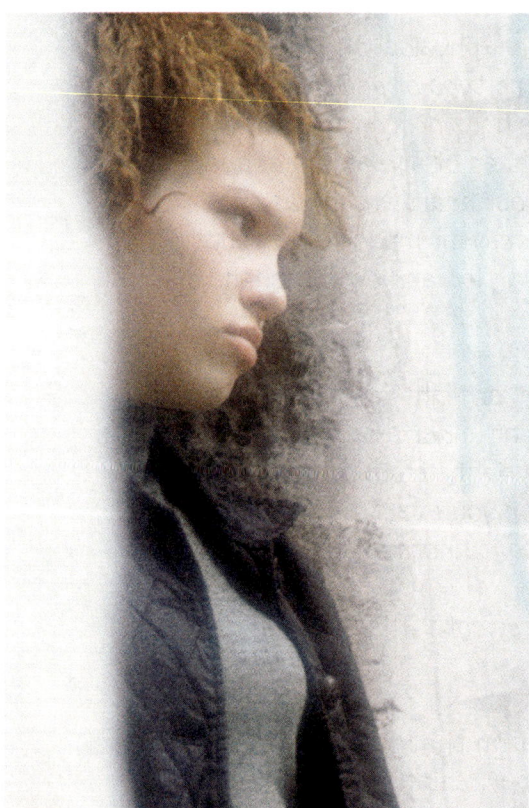

7-13 For some, depression is an effect of prolonged stress. Seeking help can lower the stress level.

Ways to Reduce Stress

It is impossible to live without stress. All people experience some stress in their lives. It is possible, however, to keep stress manageable most of the time. You can do much to reduce your stress level.

When you notice yourself getting stressed, start to make changes to relieve the stress. Find ways to help you deal better with the circumstances. If you ignore stress when it starts to build, it may have much more serious effects. This can cause you more problems than if you took care of the problem right away.

Taking a deep breath is one of the easiest ways to reduce feelings of stress. It helps move extra oxygen to your brain and muscles. A deep breath can also help you relax. Often all it takes to lower your stress is to relax for a little while. Even if this doesn't take the stress away, you'll feel more prepared to handle it if you can relax for a while.

Other ways to relax vary from person to person. Taking time to do an activity you enjoy can be relaxing. For some, this will be listening to favorite music or sounds of nature. Others find physical activity helps them relax. Stretching exercises or yoga may decrease tension in your muscles. Walking or doing aerobics may relax you. Still other people like drawing, writing in a journal, or doing crafts. Do an activity you find relaxing. This can take your mind off your problems and help you leave stress behind.

Feeling confident in your decision-making skills can also reduce stress. Knowing you made the right choice can be a relief. (Refer again to Chapter 3 to review the steps of the decision-making process.) Consistently using these steps to solve problems may lower your stress level.

If stress starts to control your life, you may want to seek help. Sometimes just talking to someone about it is all it takes. You might talk with your parents, friends, religious leader, or caseworker. Teachers and counselors might also be good listeners. They may be able to help you find solutions to your stressors. You may also be able to call a teen talk line. The volunteers who answer the phone are trained to talk to teens about their concerns.

Ways to Prevent Stress

Some stressors can't be eliminated. For instance, you may not be able to avoid dealing with child support issues, court dates, and public aid. Other stressors can be prevented, though. You can try to stay out of the grocery store at its busiest time. You can also leave early enough to get to places on time without rushing. By ridding your life of unnecessary stress, you will find the rest of it more manageable.

First, you can prevent stress by managing your time. When you plan ahead, you can avoid schedule conflicts. You can prioritize and choose the activities that matter most to you. This will reduce tension and confusion about what you will be doing.

By managing your time, you can also find time for yourself. Doing activities you like is important. Taking care of yourself matters, too. You can maintain or improve your health by eating well, staying active, and resting enough. See Figure 7-14. This will help you be at your best to meet the challenges you will face.

When you feel refreshed, you may not interpret as many events as stressful. Instead, you might see them as minor annoyances you can easily overcome. Your attitude and point of view have much to do with the stress you feel. If you can keep a positive outlook, you will be much happier and feel less stress. When you let things worry you, the tension will rise.

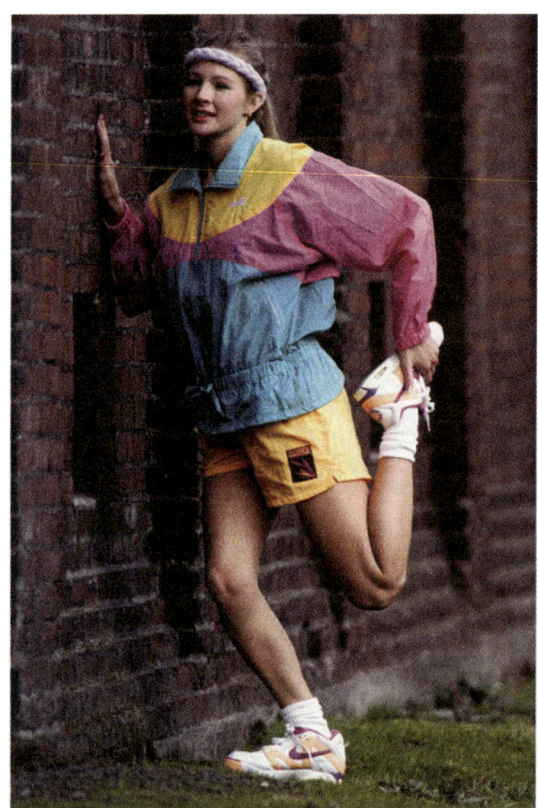

7-14 Staying active will help you prevent and manage stress.

One final way to prevent stress is to stop expecting perfection in everything you do. You may be expecting too much from yourself. You are only one person and can only do so much. It is important to accept this fact. Since you can't do everything perfectly, you may need to choose some areas in which you can lower your expectations of yourself. For instance, you might cut back your hours at work. You might be satisfied with a B instead of an A on some schoolwork. A perfectly neat home might not be your goal. You might turn down an activity that would crowd your schedule and make you stressed.

By paying attention to your stress, you can learn how to prevent or reduce it. Managing your stress in a healthful way can help you enjoy life more. This will benefit both you and your child.

Major Points

- As a teen, your main task is to prepare for adulthood. When you became a parent, this added a new and important role. Your main task as a parent is to provide care and guidance for your child. These two roles can conflict, causing you to feel overwhelmed.

- Your baby will demand much of your time and attention. You will have to make many adjustments in your lifestyle so you can meet your child's needs. This may mean changing the way you manage your time, money, schoolwork, and job responsibilities.

- Having a baby changes your life and your relationships with others. As you take on this new role, you will form new expectations of others. What they expect of you will change, too. Communication will help your relationships adjust positively to the changes.

- Teen parents may feel stress for many reasons. Pressures regarding time, money, parenting concerns, school, work, and relationships are the most common causes. Identifying common stressors in your life is the first step to getting stress under control.

- Stress can affect the body in a number of different ways. Prolonged stress can harm both your physical and emotional health. For this reason, it's important to find ways to reduce or control the stress in your life.

Chapter 8 Relationships and Sexual Decision Making

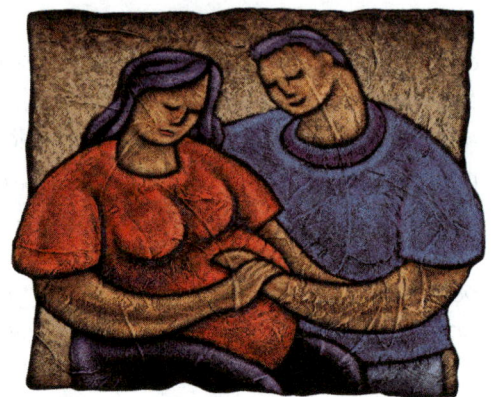

After having a baby, you have a whole new set of responsibilities. As a result of this, your relationships may change. You and your baby's other parent may still be together, or you may have broken up. You may be with someone new, or not dating anyone right now. Whatever relationship you're in now or considering in the future, make sure it's a healthy one. You and your child deserve this.

With relationships come decisions about sex. These can be tough decisions. They involve your emotions and your partner's emotions. The two of you can work together to make the best choice for your relationship. Don't be pressured to have sex because you think everyone else does. Many teens don't. Also, just because you've had sex in the past doesn't mean you must continue. You have the right to set new limits at any time. It is always your right to say no.

If you decide to have sex, make sure you're doing it for the right reasons. You and your partner must also think about the risks sex brings. The two of you need to protect yourselves from sexually transmitted infections (STIs) and unplanned pregnancy. This chapter will give you the information you need to make these tough decisions. Thinking these matters through carefully shows you are responsible.

Building a Healthy Relationship

Are you involved with someone now? If so, is this a healthy relationship? You deserve a relationship that is satisfying and rewarding. This is one that improves your life and helps you become a better person and parent. A healthy relationship is based on trust, honesty, respect, and caring. See Figure 8-1.

It's important to evaluate the health of your relationship from time to time. To do this, ask yourself the following questions about the relationship:

- Do I genuinely like my partner and feel at ease with him or her?
- Do we share many things in common?
- When we're together, do we find lots to talk about?
- Can my partner and I share our thoughts and feelings with each other?
- Do I respect my partner? Would I consider him or her a friend?

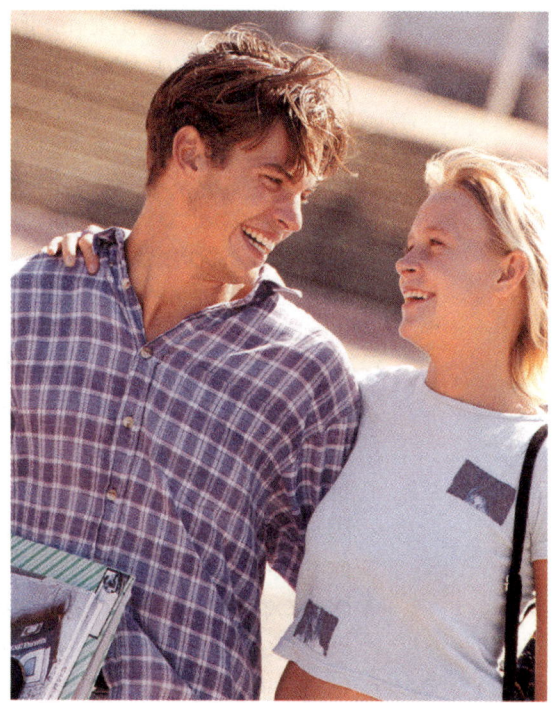

8-1 In a healthy relationship, both you and your partner can feel valued just for being yourselves.

If you can answer <u>yes</u> to these questions, you're off to a good start. You and your partner have the foundation for a good relationship. Rethink things if you answered <u>no</u> to one or more of them. If you're not with someone now, remember these points when you begin a new relationship in the future. Learning more can help you build a good relationship when the time is right.

You want to be with someone who can handle his or her emotions and express them appropriately. You need to be able to do this, too. Even when you and your partner disagree, each of you should respect the other's opinion. Neither of you should be violent, manipulative, blaming, or abusive. Each of you should have equal power and control within the relationship. You should work together to make decisions about the relationship. This includes choices about sex. Each person should take responsibility for his or her actions and accept the results of them.

Choose a relationship that allows you to keep growing as a person. Each of you needs to reach goals, develop talents, and pursue interests of his or her own. Neither should be threatened by the other's success. Each of you should keep your own identity. Neither should drop your relationships with friends or family. Don't expect your partner to devote all his or her time and attention to you. By the same token, don't give up personal time, hobbies, or interests that might help you grow.

In a strong relationship, each partner sets boundaries. A *boundary* is a limit a person places on his or her behavior and the behavior he or she will accept from others. Each person also respects the limits set by the other partner. There is more than one type of boundary. A *physical boundary* is when you decide where and how someone may touch you. It means you know your comfort level and can express this to your partner in a respectful way. With an *emotional boundary*, you don't let others manipulate you by playing on your feelings. It means you won't let someone talk you into doing something for the wrong reasons. A *mental boundary* is holding onto your own thoughts and beliefs. It means not being swayed to agree with whatever the other person says. You can stand up for your beliefs and speak out when others try to persuade you. It's good to set boundaries. This tells others you value yourself and care what happens to you.

Recognizing an Unhealthy Relationship

Almost everyone wants his or her partner relationship to be healthy. Unfortunately, this isn't always the case. Some are unhealthy from the start. Others begin well but fall into problems along the way. Knowing what a good relationship is can help you spot trouble in your own relationships. You can also watch for signs your relationship may be becoming unhealthy. A list of these is given in Figure 8-2.

Do you notice one or more of these problems in your relationship? If so, think about what you and your partner could do to fix the problem. Share your thoughts with him or her. Find out what your partner thinks about the issue. Suppose he or she denies there is a problem or is unwilling

What Can Make a Relationship Unhealthy?

Relationships can become unhealthy for many reasons. Below are a few examples of situations that might cause this to happen. Problems can occur when either partner

- has different expectations of the relationship than the other partner (examples: one person wants to marry while the other wants casual sex; one person thinks the relationship is exclusive while the other wants to "date around")
- has an addiction that interferes with the relationship (examples: drugs, alcohol, gambling)
- doesn't treat the other partner (or the partner's child) with respect
- doesn't abide by the boundaries set by the other
- abuses the other partner (or the partner's child) emotionally, physically, or sexually
- is involved in activities that are dangerous, unhealthy, or illegal (examples: being active in a gang, using or selling drugs, drinking, or stealing)
- uses the other for sex, money, possessions, or status
- shows possessive or controlling behavior
- tries to isolate the other from friends and family
- constantly argues and fights with others
- lies to, cheats on, or steals from the other partner
- focuses too much on sexual part of the relationship
- has unresolved personal problems that affect his or her ability to be involved in a healthy relationship (examples: serious family issues, past relationship issues, eating disorders or addictions, low-self esteem, severe depression, unresolved grief)
- settles for an unsatisfying relationship to avoid being alone
- feels scared of or intimidated by the other partner
- is afraid to share honest thoughts, feelings, and needs with the other—keeps problems to himself or herself to avoid losing the relationship or angering the other person
- allows the other person to continually take advantage of him or her
- focuses solely on pleasing the other

 8-2 Are any of these situations present in your relationship? What other signs might indicate an unhealthy relationship?

to change. What do you think this means for your relationship? What would you do if your partner wants you to change in ways that aren't acceptable to you?

Suppose your relationship concerns are caused by your unresolved problems. You might not have gotten over your feelings about becoming a parent so soon. Past or current family problems may be affecting your relationship with your partner. Resolving these personal issues will help you grow as a person. This will help you be able to give more fully to a relationship.

It can be hard to admit your relationship is unhealthy. Ignoring the problems only makes them worse, though. The sooner you handle the situation, the better you will probably feel. Sometimes this means breaking things off. Ending an unhealthy relationship would free each of you to find someone with whom you're a better match. It can be sad to end a relationship, but that's better than staying in one that isn't good for you or makes you unhappy. You and your child deserve to be treated well. If your partner's behavior is putting you or your child in danger or at risk, leave the relationship as soon as possible. You and your child deserve to be safe.

If you need help deciding what to do about your relationship, you might want to see a counselor. He or she could help you work through your feelings and decide what will be best for you and your child.

Making Responsible Sexual Decisions

Part of a relationship is deciding how you and your partner will show your feelings for each other. This includes decisions about whether you and your partner will have sex. These choices can be tough to make, but they're important. The results can affect the rest of your life. Making a responsible decision will keep you from rushing into something for which you're not ready or really don't want.

Each person has personal values and beliefs that will guide choices about sex. The factors involved with this decision differ for each person. Consider someone who is dating, someone in a serious relationship, and someone who's married. Each person's situation has unique factors and concerns. After having a baby, your choices about sex may be much more involved than before.

Many people feel sex should be reserved for marriage. Most faiths discourage having sex outside the marital relationship. To many people, sex is a sacred and intimate act. They believe it should be shared only by people who have made the commitment to share their lives together. In the context of this relationship, sex can be a meaningful way to express love. It is pleasurable and special.

Other people view sex as a casual act between two consenting people. This type of sex can satisfy physical desires, but it doesn't fulfill the other kinds of closeness most people seek from a relationship. Many people have sex when what they really want is an emotional connection. This can create a feeling of emptiness. In this kind of a relationship, sex can lose its real meaning or value.

The risks of having sex outside of marriage are also sobering. You know how much a pregnancy can change your life. Casual sex also carries a high risk of getting certain infections. These can have lasting consequences. Many young people feel having casual sex is not worth the risks. They'd rather wait until marriage and then share a sexual relationship with only one person.

You have already had sex. It may have been very enjoyable for you or you might have been disappointed by the experience. You're also familiar with some of the ways having sex can complicate your life and your relationship. You have the right to decide about having sex in the future. Just because you've had sex in the past does not mean you have to continue.

Only _you_ can choose whether having sex is right for you at this time. Give this matter some careful thought. Be sure you are making the best decision for you. Know where you stand and what you want. Set personal boundaries about sex and stick to these. Even if you're not in a relationship now, you owe it to yourself to think ahead. Decide what your limits are regarding sex. This way you'll be prepared when you start a new relationship.

When it comes to your relationship, you and your partner should make this choice together. Take the time to talk about this subject with your partner. Let him or her know where you stand on this issue. Find out what his or her limits are, too. Don't cross your boundaries or ask your partner to cross his or hers. Within these limits, decide with your partner what will be best for your relationship.

Factors to Consider

When making decisions about sex, there are many factors to consider. Some of these involve you, your family, and your child. Others focus on your partner and your relationship with him or her. Thinking through all these factors will help you and your partner make responsible choices about sexual behavior.

As with all decisions, your choices about sex will have consequences. You need to think carefully about these consequences. How could they change your life? Be sure you can live with the consequences of the actions you choose. See Figure 8-3.

Start by reflecting on your values. These are your beliefs, feelings, and ideas about what is important. What do you value in life? What specific values do you have related to sexuality? See Figure 8-4. When is it okay to have sex, and with whom? What do your religious beliefs say about having sex? Think about how well each option would fit with your values. If you choose an option that conflicts with your values, you're likely to end up feeling disappointed with yourself. Choosing an option that supports your values can boost your self-esteem.

Sexual Decision Making: Factors to Consider

In order to make a responsible decision about sex, there are several factors you need to consider. Some of these include the following:

- your values and your family's values
- your life goals
- your child's needs
- your emotional readiness
- the basis of your relationship
- your feelings for your partner
- your partner's feelings for you
- your partner's values, life goals, and boundaries
- how a repeat pregnancy or STI would change your life, your partner's life, and your families' lives

8-3 Responsible sexual decision making involves considering your options in terms of many important factors.

Second, think about your family's values. You're mature enough to have many of your own values, but your family has taught you many things. Your parents may have taught you many lessons through discussions about sexuality. They may have taught just as much (or more) by example. Does your family believe sex should be limited to marriage? Do they believe sex is okay if the two people are committed to each other? Consider these values as you decide when to have a sexual relationship again. If you go against your parents' beliefs, it may create a barrier between you and cause problems in your relationship with them. You may also have feelings of guilt. For this reason, many teens choose the option that fits within their family's values.

As you consider your readiness for a sexual relationship, think about your life goals. What are you working to accomplish now? What do you want to achieve in the next year or five years from now? How would having sex or waiting affect these goals? Choose the option that best supports your goals. Making any other choice might sabotage your plans and dreams.

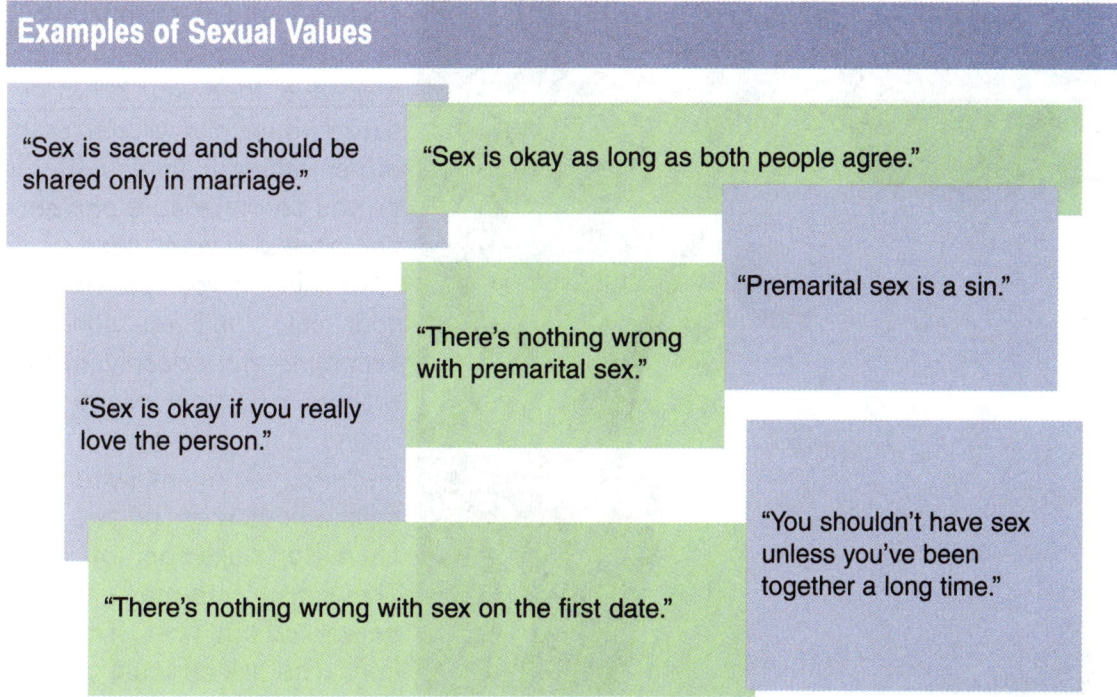

Examples of Sexual Values

"Sex is sacred and should be shared only in marriage."

"Sex is okay as long as both people agree."

"Premarital sex is a sin."

"There's nothing wrong with premarital sex."

"Sex is okay if you really love the person."

"You shouldn't have sex unless you've been together a long time."

"There's nothing wrong with sex on the first date."

8-4 Do any of these statements reflect your sexual values? Identifying your values will help you decide which option is the best decision for you.

For example, if you choose to have sex, you must accept that you might become pregnant. Using birth control can help prevent this, but it's not a guarantee. Only abstinence is 100 percent effective. Are you ready for another baby? Having a second baby now might hurt your chances of finishing school. Child care for two children is very costly. Two children are also much more work than one, especially when they are close together in age. This can mean two sets of diapers and bottles to deal with at one time. The only way to guarantee pregnancy won't occur is to choose not to have sex.

As a parent, you have your child's best interest to think about, too. No matter what you decide, you must still be available to meet your child's needs. See Figure 8-5. Will having a sexual relationship take too much time away from your child? Consider this when making your decision. You should also think about the example you'd be setting for her. What message does your behavior send? Your child will get many of her values from you. It's up to you to make sure she gets the ones you want her to have. Also, if your partner and your child don't get along, becoming more deeply involved with your partner might cause more problems. Instead, you might want to think about why the two of them don't like each other. These problems may need to be worked out first. If the concerns are serious, you should consider leaving the relationship or seeking counseling.

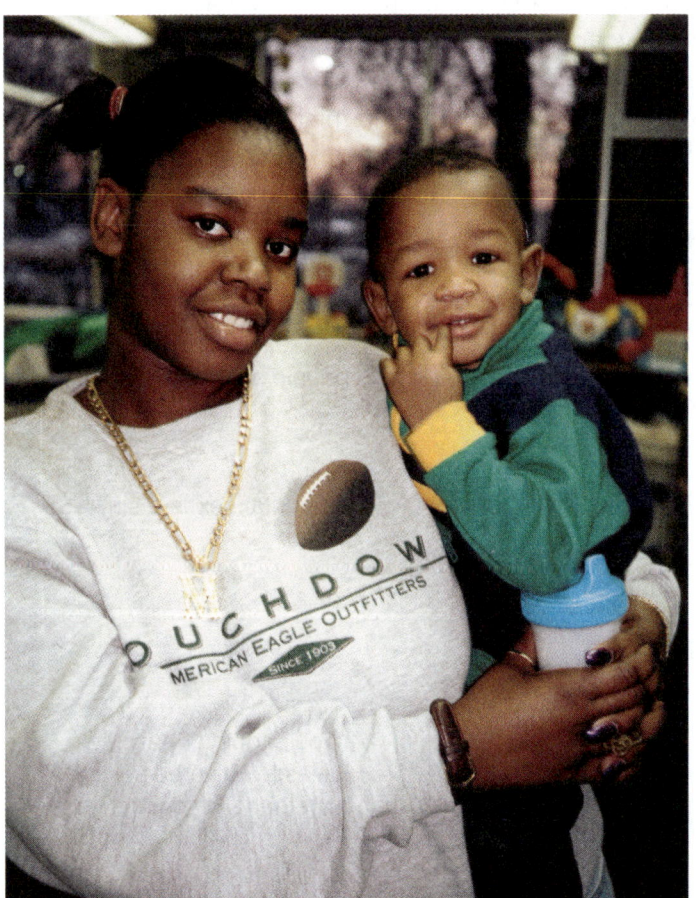

8-5 As a parent, you owe it to your child to consider his or her needs when making important decisions.

Think about your emotional readiness. Are you ready to be emotionally involved with another person to the degree sex demands? As a new parent, you've had to cope with a great deal in the past months. If you're still with your baby's other parent, how would having or not having sex now affect the relationship emotionally? If you're with someone new, are you ready to enter a sexual relationship or would it be better to wait?

A sexual relationship can create many different feelings. Some are positive, while others may not be. These emotions can be very intense. On the positive side, a sense of deep attachment may form. However, this can make it very difficult if the other person breaks up with you. Can you deal with both the pleasant and unpleasant feelings that may result from sex? Are you willing to feel the pain of loss, disappointment, and anger if the relationship ends? All these negative feelings are intensified when sex has been involved. If you wait to have sex, you can give the relationship a chance to grow. You can wait to find out if this is the right person before involving yourself sexually.

You should also consider the basis of your relationship with your partner as you make this decision. How serious and strong is the relationship? What would having (or not having) sex add to it? Would sex be the focus of your relationship, or simply one small part of it? Relationships based on sex alone are not likely to be healthy or last. Would you be having sex only to keep your partner? If so, this is a warning sign. A partner who would leave you for not having sex doesn't really want to be with you anyway. He or she is more focused on having sex. This is not the kind of person you want in your life.

How long (and how well) do you really know each other? Can you trust this person and believe what he or she says? What kind of risks does your partner carry? Has he or she had partners in the past, gotten any STIs, or used IV needles to inject drugs? If this person has had past partners, has he or she been tested for STIs recently?

Finally, what are your feelings toward your partner? What are his or her feelings toward you? Can you share your feelings openly with one another? Are you in love with each other or only infatuated? Do you and your partner care about and respect one another? Will you be sensitive to each other's needs? If not, you may find entering a sexual relationship with this person is less than satisfying.

When making this decision, remember that sex does not equal love. The two are not the same. Unfortunately, some people have sex without loving their partners. They use sex only for pleasure. They want to feel good, but give nothing to their partners in return. This is not expressing love. It is sexual exploitation.

You can also love someone without having sex. A love relationship doesn't have to include sex for the feelings to be real. Sex is one way that people who genuinely love each other can express those feelings when they're ready to do so. There are many other ways to express love, too.

Choosing Abstinence

Many people decide they're not ready to have a sexual relationship. They choose not to have sex, an option that is called abstinence. Choosing abstinence doesn't mean deciding you will never have sex again. It means choosing to postpone sex until you're ready to enter this type of relationship. You can be abstinent now even if you've had a sexual relationship in the past.

Abstinence has many benefits. This choice can protect your future goals, plans, and dreams. It can keep you from being swept up in a relationship that turns out to be unsatisfying. Abstinence will protect you from unplanned pregnancies and STIs. See Figure 8-6. Avoiding these consequences can allow you to focus on other aspects of life, such as parenting, school, and personal growth. Waiting to have sex can help you build a stronger relationship with your partner first. It can protect you emotionally and physically until you're ready to enter a sexual relationship.

These benefits lead many teens to choose abstinence. This number is growing as more teens realize what they have to gain by waiting. These teens still date and have fun, but they maintain the boundaries they've set. Many choose to date only in groups. Others date in pairs but pick public places for their dates, such as the movies, sporting and school events, and going out to eat. In these places, it's easier to stick to their boundaries. This can be harder when a couple is alone together in a car or one partner's house for long periods of time.

If you choose abstinence, you can find other ways to express your feelings for your partner. You might hug, kiss, or hold hands. Be prepared to stick to your boundaries, though. If either of you finds this contact tempts you to go further, you may need to stop these behaviors. You can also express your feelings in words. Tell your partner how you feel or write it in a poem, song, or letter.

Make a list of things you and your partner can do instead of having sex. For example, you might participate in a sport or activity you both like. You could work on a community service project together. Work together on a hobby you both enjoy. Spend time together doing things with family and friends. You can find many ways to enjoy your relationships without having sex.

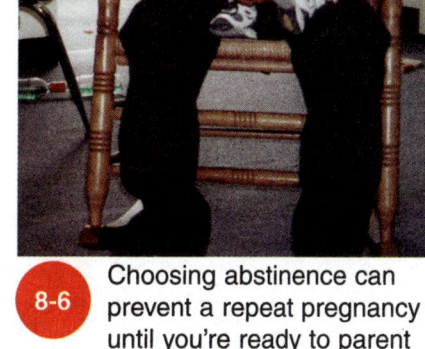

8-6 Choosing abstinence can prevent a repeat pregnancy until you're ready to parent another child.

Preventing Sexually Transmitted Infections

Did you know that every minute in the United States, an average of five teens get a sexually transmitted infection (STI)? This is an infection spread from person to person through sexual contact. Sometimes these infections are called sexually transmitted diseases (STDs).

Many health care providers feel STIs are an epidemic. Millions of people are infected each year. Most of these cases occur among people who are 15 to 24 years old. These infections can have long-lasting effects. They can damage a person's body and his or her fertility. STIs can cause discomfort, pain, or even death. Your body cannot build immunity to STIs. Even if you've had an STI in the past, you can get it again. With each sexual contact, you risk getting an STI.

Abstinence is the only way to eliminate your risk of an STI. It gives you 100 percent protection. Waiting until marriage to have sex can protect your chance to have a healthy sexual relationship. If you and your spouse have sex only with each other, you'll be safe from STIs.

No other method is guaranteed to protect you from STIs. If you choose to have sex, there are steps you can take to reduce your risk. See Figure 8-7. Following these steps can give you some protection against STIs.

Some STIs can be cured while others cannot. Each of these illnesses can harm your body and your health. The following sections describe some of the most common STIs, their symptoms, and their treatments. Learning about the risks of STIs can help you make an informed choice about whether to have sex.

Reducing Your Risk for STIs

- **Evaluate your partner's behavior.** Avoid having sex with someone you don't know well. You don't really know what type of risk this person is. Avoid having sex with a partner who won't discuss his or her sexual history, whom you suspect might cheat on you, or whom you don't feel you can trust completely and believe. Avoid a partner who is using illegal drugs. These types of partners are more likely to have (or get) an STI and hide this information from you. Having sex only with someone you know well and trust can lower your risk. Choose a partner who is open and honest with you and will be faithful to you sexually.

- **Limit your number of partners.** If you have sex with more than one person, chances are each of these partners has sex with others, too. This greatly increases your risk of being exposed to an STI. Having just one partner who only has sex with you can help keep your risk lower.

- **Use a latex condom for every type of sexual activity every time.** Latex condoms greatly reduce the risk of getting some, but not all, STIs. Other types of condoms do not offer the same type of protection. Make sure you use the condom correctly to ensure the best protection.

- **Avoid drugs and alcohol.** These substances can affect your ability to make responsible decisions. If you stay sober, you'll be much less likely to take risks with your sexual health. Be suspicious of a partner who is trying to get you drunk or high. This may mean he or she is trying to cloud your judgment so you'll agree to risky sex. Also, many STIs can be passed through the sharing of contaminated needles used to inject illegal drugs into a person's veins. Avoiding these drugs can lower your risk of getting these infections.

8-7 Only abstinence eliminates your risk for STIs, but there are ways to reduce the risk if you do choose to have sex.

HIV/AIDS

Millions of people have HIV and AIDS. You've likely heard about these illnesses because they receive a lot of attention from the media. These illnesses have very serious effects and there is no cure for them. They can be passed through sexual contact.

The human immunodeficiency (ih-myuh-noh-dee-FIH-shuhn-see) virus, also called HIV, breaks down the immune system. This is the body system that fights disease. When a person has HIV, his or her body slowly becomes less able to protect itself. He or she gets sick much easier than before. Even a cold can have serious effects on this person.

Over time, HIV progresses into a deadly disease. This is acquired immunodeficiency syndrome (AIDS). It can take many years for this to happen. The immune system becomes so weak it can't protect the person from life-threatening illnesses. At this point, AIDS develops. People with AIDS are much more likely to become seriously ill and less likely to recover. Many people with AIDS die from other diseases their bodies cannot fight.

To protect yourself from AIDS, you need to avoid contracting (getting) HIV. This virus is carried in bodily fluids. Contact with blood, semen, or vaginal secretions might occur during sexual activity. In fact, sex is the most common way HIV is spread. You can also get it from touching or sharing an intravenous (IV) needle used by someone who has the virus. Finally, mothers can pass HIV to children during pregnancy, birth, or breast-feeding. There is no evidence that air, mosquitoes, or casual contact, such as a hug, will spread HIV.

HIV/AIDS has no cure. Medicines are available, however, that can slow the progress of the virus. These medicines boost the immune system. By taking them, a person can live a longer, healthier life. Diet and exercise are also very important.

Most people with HIV do not have symptoms right away. If you're having sex, you should be tested for HIV every six months. It can be scary to wonder if you have HIV. It will be best for your health to find out as soon as possible, though. If you have HIV, you can get help right away before the illness worsens. If you don't have it, you can take steps to reduce your risk even more.

To find out if you have HIV, go to your health care provider and take a blood test. This test looks for antibodies made by the body to fight HIV. If you test positive, this means you have the antibodies in your blood. You also have the virus. Be careful not to spread HIV to anyone else. Don't have unprotected sex or share IV needles with anyone. If you test negative, this means no antibodies were found and you probably do not have HIV. There is, however, a chance you could have gotten HIV recently. Your body might not have had time to make enough antibodies for the test to detect. You should be retested in six months to be sure.

Chlamydia

Chlamydia (kluh-MIH-dee-uh) is the most common STI among teens. Sexual contact can spread the bacteria that cause this disease. Many people with chlamydia don't have any symptoms. Those who do may have any of the following:

- a burning or itching sensation
- painful urination
- whitish discharge from the penis or vagina
- lower abdominal pain

Chlamydia can be cured with antibiotics. If untreated, it can cause both men and women to become sterile. In pregnancy, a woman can pass this disease to her baby. It can cause the baby to have a serious eye, ear, or lung infection.

Gonorrhea

Another common STI is called gonorrhea (gah-nuh-REE-uh). It is caused by bacteria that are spread through sexual contact. Many people with gonorrhea have no symptoms. This is especially true of women. See Figure 8-8 for the symptoms of gonorrhea that sometimes occur.

Symptoms of Gonorrhea

Women
- yellow discharge from the vagina
- painful urination
- irritation of the vagina and cervix

Men
- creamy whitish or yellowish discharge from the penis
- painful urination
- burning sensation during urination

 Most people with gonorrhea have no sypmtoms, but any of these symptoms are possible, too.

Antibiotics can cure gonorrhea. If it is not treated, gonorrhea can cause sterility, blindness, heart damage, and arthritis. In pregnancy, this STI can cause miscarriage or stillbirth. It also raises the risk of a baby being born too soon. Women can also pass gonorrhea to their babies during delivery. This can cause the babies to have a serious eye infection that can lead to blindness.

Genital Herpes

Genital herpes (JEH-nuh-tuhl HUR-peez) is an incurable STI. It is caused by the herpes simplex virus (HSV). The virus is spread through physical contact with an infected person. Symptoms of herpes include headache, fever, aching muscles, pain when urinating, and swollen glands. The most obvious symptom, though, is small blisters that appear in the genital and rectal area or the mouth. These blisters look much like a cold sore or fever blister. They are very painful and highly contagious (easily spread to others).

After a few weeks the blisters heal, but the person still has the HSV virus. He or she will likely have repeated outbreaks of blisters in the future. Even when no sores are present, the person is contagious and can pass the disease to others. Over time, HSV may lead to certain cancers.

If a pregnant woman has herpes, her baby might get the HSV virus through the placenta before birth. This can cause miscarriage, stillbirth, or lifelong disabilities. The baby can also contract herpes by passing through the birth canal. After birth, this STI can damage the baby's eyes and brain. For this reason, cesarean delivery is often done.

A doctor can usually diagnose herpes by seeing the blisters on the genital area. Tests can be done to confirm this diagnosis. There is no known cure for the HSV virus. Medicines are available to lessen the discomfort of the outbreaks, however.

Genital Warts

Both men and women may get genital warts. These are small, hard growths in the reproductive organs, bladder, and rectum. They often cause great discomfort. Genital warts are caused by the human papilloma (pa-puh-LOH-muh) virus. This virus, also called HPV, is spread through contact with the genital warts of an infected person. This happens most often through sexual activity, but can also occur from other physical contact. There is no known cure for the HPV virus. It can take six to eight months after exposure before a person knows he or she has this STI. A doctor can examine a person to look for these warts.

Over time, these warts may spread or get larger. If they get large enough, they can block the urethra, vagina, or rectum. The warts can be surgically removed, but they will likely reoccur. The HPV virus may lead to cancer of the cervix, penis, or rectum.

Syphilis

Syphilis (SIH-fuh-luhs) is a three-stage STI that is caused by bacteria. The longer this treatable disease goes undetected, the more damage it does. During the first stage, a fairly painless sore called a chancre (SHAN-kuhr) appears at the site of the infection. In the male, this is often on the penis or anus. In a female, the sore may be inside the body (on the cervix or in the vagina). This makes it harder to detect. In a few weeks' time the chancre heals itself. The infection is still present in the body, though. The person is contagious and can pass the infection to others.

In the second stage, a person may have one or more of the following: rash, hair loss, swollen glands, sore throat, weight loss, wartlike growths, and fluid-filled sores. The person is highly contagious during this stage. Occasionally, after this stage, a person is mysteriously cured.

During the third stage, syphilis is no longer contagious. In this stage, though, it is the most destructive to a person's body. See Figure 8-9 for its possible effects.

Early detection of syphilis is important. This can be done with blood tests. If syphilis is found, it can be treated with penicillin. The sooner the disease is detected, the less damage it will do to the body.

The Effects of Late Syphilis	
❖ brain damage	❖ damage to the liver and kidneys
❖ insanity	❖ damage to the nervous system
❖ heart disease	❖ damage to blood vessels
❖ paralysis	❖ death

The effects of syphilis in the third stage are quite severe.

Hepatitis Type B

Hepatitis (heh-puh-TY-tuhs) type B is a serious virus that can cause liver damage and liver cancer. This type of hepatitis can be spread sexually. Pregnant women can also pass it to their babies during delivery. Hepatitis B can also be spread by sharing a needle, toothbrush, razor, or other item that has infected blood on it. For this reason, people must be sure when getting a tattoo or body piercing that a sterile needle will be used.

Most people with hepatitis B never even know they have it. However, this disease can stay in the body for many years. During this time, it can be passed to others. Hepatitis B has many symptoms. See Figure 8-10 for a list of these.

There is no cure for hepatitis B once a person has it. Serious cases can be treated with medication. Consulting with a health care provider is important to manage the disease.

A vaccine is available to prevent hepatitis B. Having three doses of the vaccine can protect a person for several years. During pregnancy, all women should be tested for hepatitis B. If they have the disease, their babies can be vaccinated soon after birth. This would protect the babies from getting the disease. All babies and children under age 18 should receive this vaccine. Adults who are at risk should be vaccinated, too. These include people who have had more than one sexual partner and people who use IV drugs. People who work in the health care field and might come into contact with blood or other bodily fluids should also be vaccinated.

Trichomoniasis

Trichomoniasis (trih-kuh-muh-NY-ih-suhs) is an infection that is caused by a one-celled animal called a protozoan (proh-tuh-ZOH-uhn). This infection, often called trich, is usually passed sexually. A person can get it other ways, too.

Common Symptoms of Hepatitis B

- weakness
- nausea and loss of appetite
- jaundice (yellow eyes and skin)
- dark urine
- fever
- headaches
- stomach, muscle, and joint pain

Hepatitis B is a serious disease that affects the liver. If untreated, it can even lead to death.

Most men with trich have no symptoms. When they do, these include a tingling sensation in the penis, painful urination, or a thin discharge. Women more often have symptoms from trich. These include the following:

- vaginal discharge (yellow-green or gray) with a foul odor
- itching in the genital area
- painful urination
- abdominal pain
- discomfort during sex

If trich is not treated, it can cause infections of the urethra, bladder, vagina, and cervix. A health care provider can take a sample of the discharge. Lab tests of this sample can confirm that a person has trich. To treat trich, a very strong medicine must be prescribed. A woman cannot use this medicine while she's pregnant. Both partners must be treated at the same time to be sure trich is cured.

Pubic Lice

Pubic lice are tiny gray parasites that attach to the hair of the pubic area. They are very contagious and can be passed by close physical contact, including sex. Pubic lice are sometimes called crab lice or "crabs". They lay eggs, which hatch into even more lice. These lice cause intense itching and irritation of the genital area. By looking closely, you would be able to see pubic lice and their eggs in the hair and on the skin if they were present.

If you think you have pubic lice, ask your health care provider for advice. He or she may recommend a medicated lotion or shampoo that can kill the lice. Follow the directions carefully. After all the lice and eggs have been killed, wash all the clothing, towels, sheets, and personal items that may have come into contact with them.

Scabies

Scabies (SKAY-beez) is a skin infection caused by mites. It can be spread by close physical or sexual contact. The mites burrow (dig a path) under the skin and lay eggs. This can cause itching, swelling, and a sore at the site where the mites enter the body. Scabies can be detected with a microscope. A health care provider can recommend a medicated lotion to cure it.

Vaginal Infections

Some, but not all, women have vaginal infections from time to time. This means the vagina becomes infected, swells, and causes a discharge. The vaginal area may be very painful or itchy. Vaginal infections are caused by an overgrowth of bacteria in the vagina. The most common kind of vaginal infection is a yeast infection.

The bacteria that cause these infections can be spread through sexual contact. They can also have other causes. Some of these include tight-fitting underwear or clothing; fragrances or dyes in toilet paper, soaps, douches, or bubble baths; and certain medications.

If you think you may have a vaginal infection, see your health care provider. Only he or she can tell you whether it is a vaginal infection or another STI. Your provider can tell you how to treat the infection, too. Some can be treated with over-the-counter medicines. In other cases, a prescription may be needed.

If they are not treated, vaginal infections will become worse. They can make you very uncomfortable. They can also irritate and infect your other reproductive organs. Over time, they can cause scarring, which can affect your fertility.

What to Do If You Think You Have an STI

If there is a chance you might have an STI, it's important to find out right away. If you have an STI, you will want to be treated as soon as possible. Waiting will not make things any better. If you don't have an STI, you're wasting your worry. If you do, delaying only gives the infection more time to damage your body. Even if the infection has no cure, your health care provider can advise you about your condition. There may be medicines he or she can prescribe to keep you as healthy as possible.

If you're sexually active, most health experts advise being tested every six months for STIs. Your city or county health department will offer this sort of testing. These tests may be given at little or no charge. This may depend on your income. Most health departments take patients on a first come, first served basis. You don't need an appointment. A health care provider will consult with you and provide treatment if needed. Some states require your parents to be notified before you can receive treatment, depending on your age. Call the health department before you go if you have questions about the services they provide and the costs for these services.

If you prefer to see your regular health care provider, call to make an appointment. In the office, the provider will talk to you about your symptoms and the reason you want to be tested. He or she will examine your reproductive organs. During this exam, a sample may be taken for testing. A blood sample may also be drawn. These samples will be tested by a lab to find out whether an STI is present. Your health care provider should have the test results within a few days. For an HIV test, it can take as long as two weeks. Before you leave the provider's office, ask when he or she will have the results. Ask if the provider will notify you or if you should call for the results.

If you do have an STI, see your health care provider right away to discuss treatments. If needed, your provider can refer you to a specialist who can provide additional help. If you have a treatable STI, you should not have sex while you're being treated. This keeps you from spreading the infection to your partner. If you have an STI that isn't curable, talk to your provider about the risks of you spreading the infection to a partner through sex. You will want to take every precaution so you don't pass the STI to anyone else.

When you go for STI tests, you may want to take someone with you. This might be your partner, parent, sibling, or friend. This person's support can help you face this scary task. Your support person may help you think of important questions to ask during the visit. He or she can also comfort you if you're upset by the news you receive.

Learning you have an STI is stressful. At first, you may be in disbelief. You may be angry or wonder why this has happened to you. You may be sad or scared about what this means for your future. Talk to someone about these feelings. Give yourself some time to adjust to the news.

It's important to tell your sexual partner or partners about the STI. This is true as well for any past partners who might have been exposed. It can be difficult to have this discussion, but you need to do it. Your partner deserves to know if he or she was exposed to an STI. Tell your partner to get tested and treated. Otherwise, if he or she has the infection, it can be spread to others. Even if you've been cured, you could get it again from your partner unless he or she is treated.

It's also important to learn how to lower your risk of getting an STI in the future. Take care of yourself and your health. You owe it to yourself and your child.

Preventing a Repeat Pregnancy

After the birth of your child, you can become pregnant again right away. Once your body releases an egg, pregnancy can occur. There is no way to tell when your body will start to release eggs again. It will happen before your period returns, even if you're breast-feeding. This creates a risk of repeat pregnancy. If you choose to be sexually active, you need to decide how you will handle this risk.

A repeat pregnancy creates many health risks. Pregnancy and delivery put many physical demands on your body. Your body needs time to recover. You need to rest and regain your strength. Your body must start to rebuild the nutrient stores that were depleted during pregnancy. It may take as long as 18 months for your health to fully return to normal. See Figure 8-11.

When pregnancies occur too close together, it doesn't give a woman's body time to recover from the first birth. This makes complications very likely. Both the woman and her unborn child are at serious risk. This risk is even higher for teen moms. This is because their bodies are still growing and maturing. A second pregnancy in the teen years could also interfere with a young woman's own growth and development. By planning enough time between your pregnancies, you can reduce these risks.

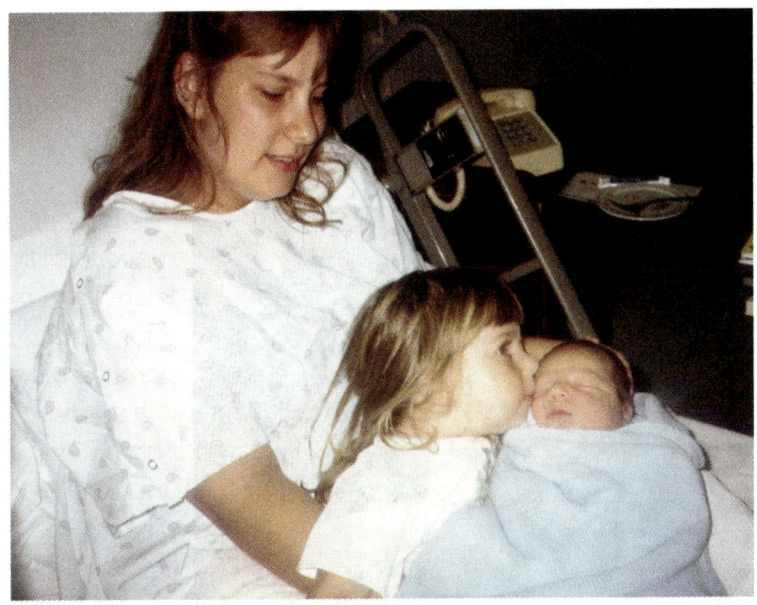

Bonnie Mori

8-11 Healing from pregnancy and delivery takes time. Spacing your pregnancies at least 18 months apart is best for your body and your next baby's health.

These health risks are not the only good reasons to wait. A repeat pregnancy brings with it many other concerns, too. Adjusting to a new routine is tiring. Getting to know your baby and learning to care for him takes time. At first, this task will be pretty demanding. Your child needs your time and attention. Being up at night for feedings can keep you from getting the rest you need. The time you must devote to feeding, bathing, dressing, and cuddling him can overwhelm you.

Becoming pregnant again right away would make things even harder. It would force you to stretch your time and energy even farther. You would have to fit in two baths, two sets of feedings and changes, and twice as much cuddling time. All these tasks would have to be squeezed into your already full schedule.

Having a child is very expensive. Having two children costs even more. Child care costs for two children can be especially costly. Is there room in your budget to take on these additional costs? Can you afford another child right now?

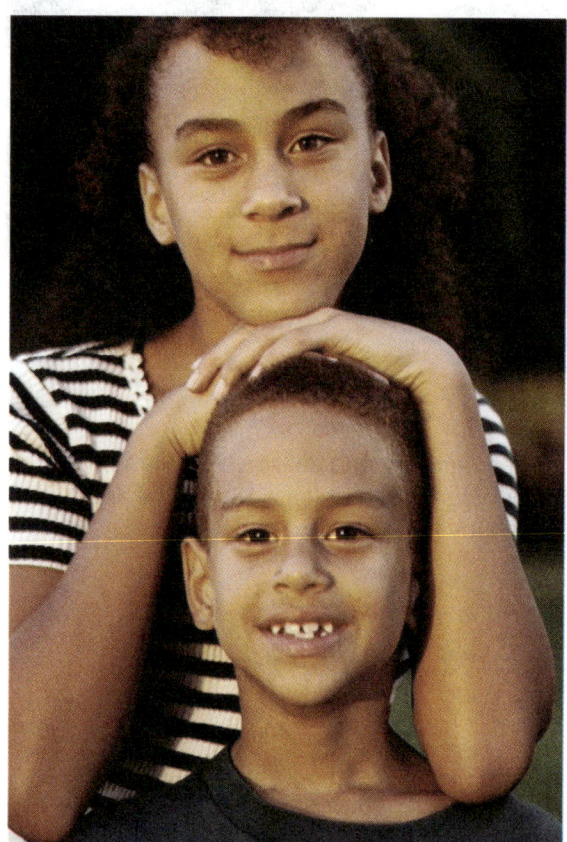

8-12 Children often experience less sibling rivalry when they're spaced two to three years apart.

For some teen parents, the extra responsibility of a second child can keep them from meeting their goals. Studies show having a second child makes teen parents more likely to drop out of school. It also makes them more likely to rely on public aid. Postponing your next pregnancy until you've met some of your life goals will give you and your children a better life. It will help you feel better about yourself. Finishing school will also increase your earning power. This will help you meet the added costs if you choose to have a second child.

Finally, studies show children do best when spaced two to three years apart. This much time lets each child achieve a separate status in the family. It reduces sibling rivalry, or strong competitive and jealous feelings between brothers and sisters. A child who is at least two years old is less likely to feel replaced as the baby of the family when a new child comes along. See Figure 8-12.

Contraceptive Methods

A contraceptive (kahn-truh-SEHP-tihv) is any method a couple uses to keep the woman from conceiving. These methods prevent the union of egg and sperm. Their purpose is to prevent pregnancy. Some of these methods supply hormones to keep a woman's body from releasing an egg. Other methods provide a barrier between the sperm and egg. This makes it impossible for them to meet.

Abstinence

Abstinence is the <u>only</u> method that is 100 percent effective against pregnancy and STIs. Most religions view this as the best choice until marriage. It allows you to focus on your life goals. Having a second baby now would only complicate your life. Getting an STI would, too.

You've already had sex, but you can decide to start abstaining now. Many teens choose this option. It is sometimes called *secondary virginity*. Abstinence can help you keep life simple until you're ready for a sexual relationship again. Many teen parents feel this will be in the future when they are married.

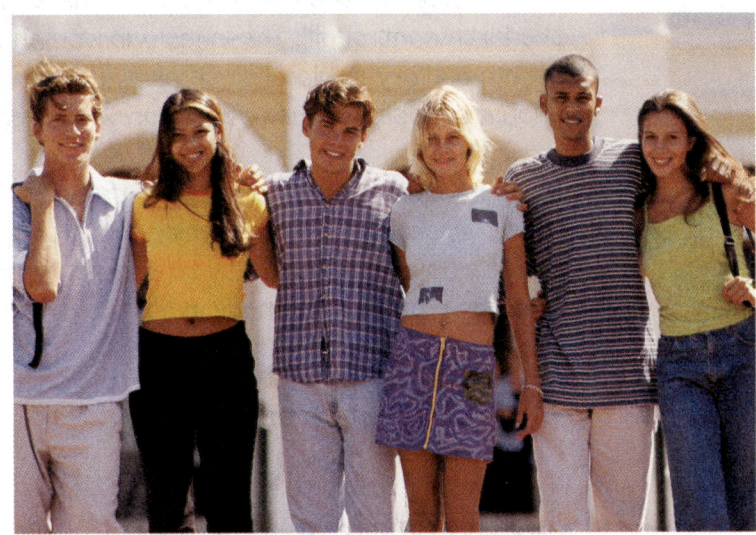

8-13 Group dates allow teens to have fun dating while still honoring their boundaries.

To make this method work, you must be committed to it. You will need to avoid situations that might tempt you to change your mind. This may mean more public dates and less private time with your partner. See Figure 8-13. Since this decision will affect both of you, it's best to discuss this with him or her. Be clear about your boundaries and your reasons for setting them. If your partner can't respect your choice, perhaps it's time to reconsider whether he or she is the right person for you.

Birth Control Pills

The *birth control pill* is a daily hormone pill that prevents pregnancy. Its hormones keep a woman's body from releasing an egg. The birth control pill is prescribed by a health care provider. It must be taken at the same time each day. When used correctly, the pill is 92 to 99 percent effective against pregnancy. Incorrect use can cause this method to fail.

Since it is a hormonal method, the birth control pill does not offer any protection against STIs. It also causes side effects in some women. Mild side effects include breast tenderness, headaches, depression, and weight gain. Talk to your health care provider about more serious side effects.

Because of the side effects, some women are advised not to use the birth control pill. These include women who smoke, are obese, or have a history of blood clots or high blood pressure. These women should choose another way to prevent pregnancy.

Certain medicines and herbs can interfere with the pill's effectiveness. Antibiotics, which are often used to treat infections, can disrupt the pill's ability to prevent pregnancy. When a health care provider prescribes a medicine for you, let him or her know if you take the birth control pill.

Contraceptive Injection

Another method is the contraceptive injection (shot). A health care provider gives it in the buttock or upper arm. Its purpose is to prevent pregnancy. A health care provider will explain how long it will work, usually several weeks or months. The injection contains a synthetic hormone that prevents a woman's egg cells from being released. Bleeding, missed periods, breast pain, weight gain, headaches, and nausea sometimes occur with this injection. This method is 97 percent effective.

Skin Patch

Health care providers may prescribe a skin patch. It looks like a bandage and is less than two inches long. The woman attaches it to her lower stomach, buttocks, or upper body. It should never be placed on the breast. It releases hormones into the bloodstream. The skin patch can prevent pregnancy if a new patch is applied each week for a total of three weeks. She does not use the patch during the fourth week, so she can have her menstrual period. The patch has risks similar to other hormonal forms of birth control. One disadvantage of this method can be skin irritation. Another disadvantage is if the patch comes off before the end of the week. This method is 98 to 99 percent effective.

Vaginal Contraceptive Ring

Another method that releases hormones is the vaginal contraceptive ring. It is a flexible, transparent ring that must be prescribed by a doctor. It is placed in the vagina where it releases hormones that prevent the egg from being fertilized. This method is 92 percent effective. The woman can insert and remove the ring, making it more convenient than going to the doctor. When in contact with the woman's vagina, it continually releases a low dose of hormones. As with the skin patch, she uses it for three weeks. She then removes it for one week in order to start her menstrual period. After the fourth week, she inserts a new ring into her vagina to continue the process. If the ring moves out of place during activities, including sexual intercourse, it must be replaced within three hours. This will keep it effective. If it is not replaced within three hours, a backup birth control method is needed until a new ring has been in place for seven days.

Spermicide

A spermicide is a chemical that kills sperm or makes them unable to swim to the egg. Spermicide comes in many forms. These include foams, creams, jellies, films, and tablets.

Spermicide can be used alone, but it is only 74 percent effective when used this way. A better use is to combine it with other methods. Some condoms have spermicide added to them. Both the diaphragm and cervical cap require the use of spermicide. It can also be used with hormonal methods such as the birth control pill.

Spermicide is sold over the counter and may be purchased without a prescription. To be effective, it must be applied with each sexual act. How these products are used depends on their form and whether they're used alone or combined with another method. Read the instructions or ask a health care provider for advice.

Condoms

A condom is a thin sheath that fits over the erect penis. The semen (which contains sperm) collects in the end of the condom. This keeps it from going into the vagina. Condoms can be bought in many places, such as grocery stores, drugstores, and convenience stores. Some vending machines even offer condoms for sale. Each condom is used once and thrown away. Never reuse a condom.

The condom's effectiveness against pregnancy is about 88 percent. This depends mostly on correct use. Even when used correctly, a condom can fail. It may tear, break, or slip off the penis. For added protection, choose a condom with spermicide or add spermicide to the condom before using it. If you need a lubricant, choose one that is water-based. Petroleum-based products can break down the rubber in the condom, causing it to tear.

Condoms are made of latex, polyurethane (pah-lee-YUHR-ih-thayn), or lambskin. Most condoms are latex rubber. Except for abstinence, the latex condom offers the most protection against STIs. See Figure 8-14. It keeps the sexual organs of the male and female from coming into contact. Lambskin condoms are not recommended. This kind of condom has tiny holes in it that can allow an STI to pass through. Polyurethane condoms are fairly new. More research needs to be done on their effectiveness against STIs and pregnancy.

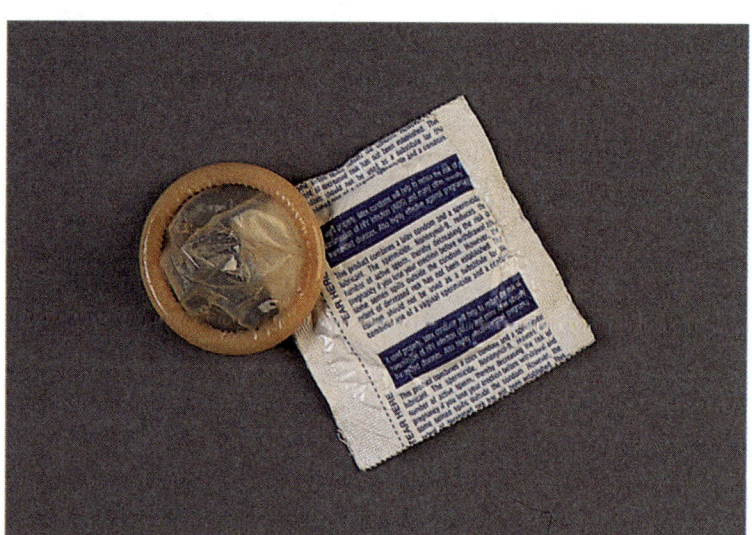

8-14 The latex condom provides more STI protection than any other birth control method.

Proper storage of condoms is important. They should be kept in a cool, dry place. If kept in a warm place, such as a wallet or car glove compartment, the latex slowly breaks down, causing the condom to fail. Also, check the condom wrapper for an expiration date before using. Over time, the latex can become dry and brittle, causing the condom to break. For this reason, do not use an expired condom.

<u>Even if you use another contraceptive, it's good to use a latex condom, too</u>. This increases your protection against pregnancy and STIs. It can give you more peace of mind.

A female condom is also available. It is made of polyurethane and has two rigid rings. One fits around the cervix and the other hangs outside the vagina. The female condom prevents pregnancy in only 74 percent of cases. It provides some STI protection, but it is not known exactly how much. Like the male condom, it can only be used once and then thrown away. The female condom is not available in as many places as the male version. It also costs much more.

Diaphragm

The diaphragm (DY-uh-fram) is a thin rubber cup with a rigid rim. It covers the woman's cervix and acts as a barrier. The diaphragm keeps sperm from reaching the egg. It must be fitted by a health care provider. This is because the diaphragm must be exactly the right size to fit the woman's body and prevent pregnancy. Unless it is damaged, the diaphragm can be used for up to a year before being replaced. It is about 84 to 94 percent effective for preventing pregnancy.

The diaphragm is inserted before intercourse. Spermicide must be applied to it before use. Within two hours before intercourse, the woman inserts the diaphragm. It can be left in for as long as 24 hours. The diaphragm itself does not protect against STIs, but the spermicide used with it offers some STI protection.

After having a baby, a woman may not be able to use the same diaphragm she used before she was pregnant. Pregnancy, labor, and delivery may have changed the shape of her cervix slightly. Her health care provider should check the fit of her diaphragm. A new diaphragm of a different size may be needed.

Cervical Cap and Cervical Shield

The cervical cap and cervical shield are similar to the diaphragm. The cervical cap is shaped like a thimble. A cervical shield is a similar device that has an air valve and loop to aid in removal. Both are designed to firmly cover the opening of the cervix and act as a barrier to sperm, preventing them from entering the uterus. A health care provider must fit these devices because their measurements must be exact. They must be used with spermicide and inserted before intercourse. They can remain in the vagina for as long as three days.

The cervical cap and cervical shield do not protect against STIs. When used correctly (before first pregnancies), the cervical cap is 84 to 91 percent effective, and the cervical shield is 85 percent effective. After childbirth or a significant weight change, a health care provider must refit the devices.

Contraceptive Sponge

The contraceptive sponge is a small round device made of polyurethane foam. The sponge is moistened with water and placed inside the woman's vagina against the cervix. It is meant for one-time use and discarded after use. The sponge is inserted before intercourse and should remain in place at least eight hours after intercourse to be effective.

The sponge serves as a barrier that prevents sperm from entering the cervix. It also contains spermicide to prevent sperm from reaching the egg. The effectiveness of the sponge depends on whether it is used correctly. It can be anywhere from 84 to 91 percent effective (before first pregnancies). The spermicide in the sponge provides a small level of protection from STIs. The contraceptive sponge can be purchased over the counter.

Natural Family Planning

In natural family planning (also called periodic abstinence), a couple uses one of a few ways to determine when the woman is most likely to be fertile. They use this information to plan times for intercourse. To prevent pregnancy, the couple would abstain from intercourse during the most fertile days. To conceive, they would have intercourse on these days.

A health care provider can tell a couple how to predict the fertile days. This is based on the woman's menstrual cycle. Even when used correctly, these methods work only 80 percent of the time. For teens, the percentage is even lower. This is because teens often have less regular cycles, which makes mistakes more likely. For this reason, teens are advised not to use natural family planning methods.

IUD

An intrauterine (ihn-truh-YOO-tur-ihn) device (IUD) is a small, flexible plastic device. A health care provider inserts this device into the uterus to prevent pregnancy. It remains in the uterus for one to eight years (depending on the type). Use of this device was quite common 30 years ago but now is rare. The IUD is 99 percent effective, but it has many drawbacks. The most serious is the risk of the device tearing the uterus. The IUD also provides no protection against STIs. Due to these risks, teens are rarely advised to use the IUD.

Sterilization

Sterilization is the use of surgery to prevent conception. This method keeps the egg and sperm from uniting. The person's body no longer provides eggs or sperm for reproduction. If the surgery is successful, pregnancy can no longer occur.

Vasectomy (vuh-SEHK-tuh-mee) is the name for sterilization of a male. This surgery blocks a man's vas deferens (the tube that carries sperm to the penis). Blocking the tubes keeps the sperm from entering the semen. During intercourse, the man can still ejaculate, but no sperm will be released.

Tubal ligation (too-buhl LY-gay-shuhn) is the name for sterilization of a female. This surgery blocks a woman's fallopian tubes so eggs cannot travel to the uterus. Blocking the tubes keeps the eggs from being available to be fertilized by sperm. Pregnancy cannot occur.

Sterilization is considered to be permanent. Even surgery can't always reverse these methods. For this reason, sterilization is not advised for teens. Even if you don't want a pregnancy to occur now, you may change your mind several years from now. This is too permanent a choice for you to make this early in your life.

Deciding About Contraception

After the birth of your baby, you'll likely face some choices about sex. You will want to consider the risks of having sex. If you're in a relationship now, how will you and your partner handle these risks? What method will you use? The two of you might have made this choice during your pregnancy. If not, now is the time to decide.

Both you and your partner will be affected by this decision. Work together to make the best choice for your relationship. It may not be easy to talk about contraceptives, but it's important. Ignoring this issue can have long-lasting results. You show you're responsible when you discuss these risks and form a plan to prevent them.

Let your partner know what you want and expect. As you think about each option, find answers to the questions in Figure 8-15. The decision-making process can also guide you as you make this decision. (To review this process, refer to Chapter 3.)

Suppose you're not in a relationship now. It's still wise to think about preventing pregnancy. You may start dating again sooner than you think. Consider the options. Decide where you stand on this issue and what method you'd prefer. Before you have sex again, make a commitment to talk to your partner about these issues. This will protect both of you from unwanted risks.

Questions to Ask: Contraceptive Methods
- How frequently (if at all) will we have sex?
- How committed are we to using this method?
- Will my partner and I be comfortable using this method?
- Will this method help prevent STIs?
- How effective is it?
- How long does its protection last?
- Are there any side effects? Can my partner and I accept these?
- What would my partner and I need to do to use this method?
- Can my partner and I afford this method?

8-15 You and your partner can consider these questions when deciding how you'll prevent a repeat pregnancy.

Major Points

- As a teen parent, you've taken on new responsibilities. In light of these responsibilities, you need to reevaluate your partner relationship. Is this a healthy relationship for you? How does it affect your child?

- Knowing what a healthy relationship is can help you recognize an unhealthy one. If your relationship is unhealthy, you should decide whether changes can be made to improve it. If not, you should consider ending the relationship.

- With relationships come decisions about sex. You should decide whether it's best for you to keep having sex or to choose abstinence at this time. For many teen parents, postponing sex has many benefits and protects their life goals. There are many factors to consider as you make this decision. Carefully thinking the matter through is a responsible approach to sexual decision making.

- Sexual decision making also means deciding how to prevent sexually transmitted diseases (STIs). These diseases damage a person's body and his or her fertility. They can cause discomfort, pain, or even death. Each STIs has unique symptoms, effects, and treatments. Some can be cured, while others will be with a person for life. Abstinence is the only way to guarantee you will stay free from these diseases.

- Preventing a repeat pregnancy is important, too. Becoming pregnant again now might jeopardize your health and the health of your unborn baby. It would also create even more responsibilities for you to handle. Abstinence is the only guaranteed way to prevent a pregnancy. If you do choose to have sex, though, you and your partner should talk about which method of contraception you will use.

Chapter 9 Communicating for Better Relationships

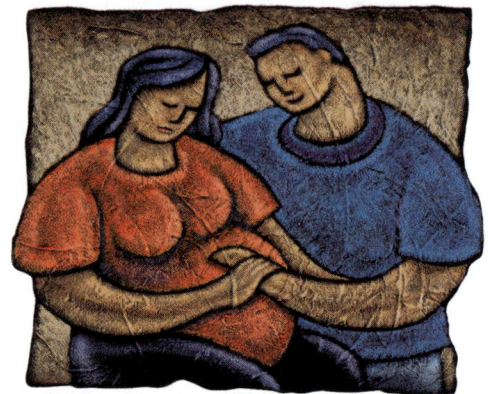

Communication is the act of exchanging messages. Each day you communicate almost constantly with friends, teachers, family members, strangers, and even pets. Communication includes both sending messages and receiving them. This two-way process is like a street on which cars go both directions. In communication, messages go back and forth between you and others.

Why is communication so important? It is the key to relationships. Can you imagine spending time with a person and never talking or using body language? Neither of you would get to know the other well. You couldn't share your thoughts, feelings, or experiences. You wouldn't know what the other person was thinking or feeling, either. It wouldn't really be a relationship.

How you communicate affects how well you will get along with others. Sending clear messages and receiving messages as they were meant is very important. By trying to make your message easy to understand for the listener, you can increase the chance the message will get through as you intended.

Good communication also means a message is correctly interpreted. Have you ever opened a package to find the instructions are written in a language you can't read? The message is there. It was correctly sent, but you can't interpret it. The same thing can happen between family members or friends. It can also happen between you and your baby. For instance, your baby may cry and cry. You try to feed, diaper, rock, pat, and comfort her, and yet she keeps crying. From her cry, you know something is wrong. The baby is sending you the correct message. You may not know how to interpret the message correctly, though. This can make you feel frustrated and helpless. It can make your baby feel misunderstood and frantic.

Key Elements of Communication

Learning more about communication can help you build your skills in sending and receiving messages. Have you ever played the game of Gossip? In this game, players sit in a line or a circle. The first person whispers a message into the ear of the second person. This person whispers the message as he or she heard it to the next person. This continues until everyone has received the message. The last person repeats to the group the message he or she heard. The final message is never the same as the original one. Why does this happen? This is simply because most people don't have perfect communication skills.

Types of Communication

Two basic types of communication are verbal and nonverbal. Verbal communication is the use of words to send or receive a message. These messages are sent by speaking or writing. They are received by hearing or reading. E-mails, letters, books, speeches, and phone calls are examples. Sign language and Braille are other examples. The signs and symbols used represent the words in the message being sent.

Nonverbal communication is the use of body language to send a message. This type of communication includes tone of voice, eye contact, gestures, facial expressions, posture, and body movements. See Figure 9-1. For instance, you may use your hands and arms to stress a point. You may smile

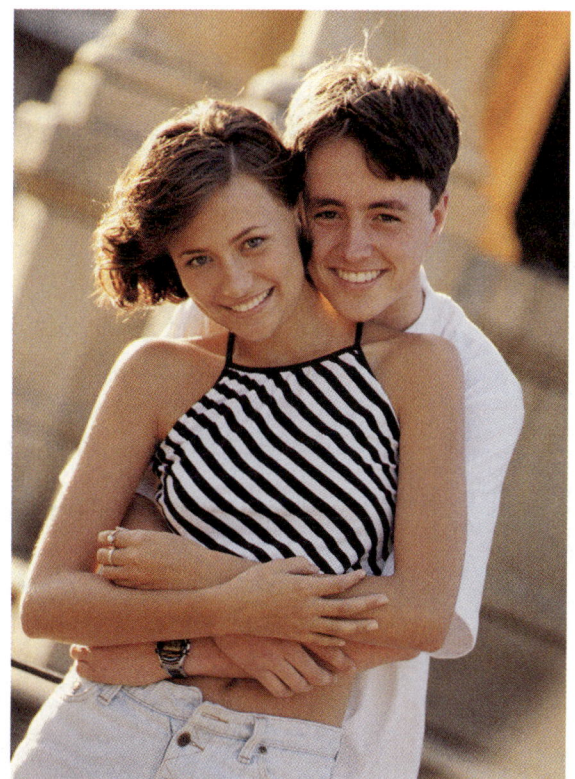

9-1 A hug can express feelings of closeness. It is a type of nonverbal communication.

or frown. You may avoid eye contact. Support or friendship can be expressed through a hug. Standing up straight can show confidence, but slouching does not. Nonverbal communication can sometimes reveal more than words.

Sometimes verbal and nonverbal messages conflict. For instance, your tone of voice may defy your words. If you scowl and shout, "Of course I love you," your verbal and nonverbal messages don't agree. In these cases, a person will often believe your nonverbal message instead of the verbal one.

Active Listening

When you communicate with friends and family, you also need to listen to what they're saying. Your purpose may be to understand their feelings. It may be to learn the reasoning behind a decision. It's important to listen rather than just hearing what is said.

In *active listening*, the listener focuses on the message and shows he or she understands it. Active listening lets the person sending the message know it has been understood. It tells the listener he or she interpreted the message correctly. Active listening prevents misunderstandings.

Taking the time to really listen shows you care about what the other person is saying. It encourages the other person to listen to you in the same way. There are several ways in which you can show you're an active listener. By practicing these skills, you can become better at interpreting the messages people send.

Maintain Eye Contact

Good listening involves eye contact. Look into the speaker's eyes when he or she talks. This is important with people of all ages. When your baby coos, eye contact tells her you're paying attention. Eye contact helps when talking with your friends and adults, too. It shows the other person's message matters to you. See Figure 9-2.

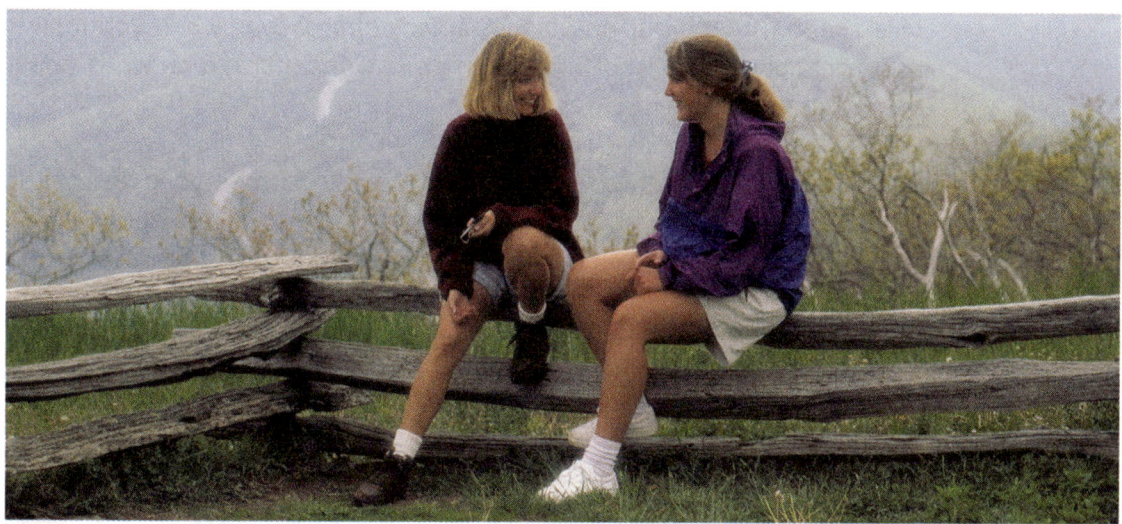

9-2 Eye contact is an essential part of active listening. It helps you focus on the speaker and shows you're paying attention.

Block out Interruptions

Active listeners focus on what the other person is saying. Sometimes this means turning off the radio or TV. It could mean moving to a quieter place. Interruptions are common when people are talking. They are also rude. A good listener lets the other person finish talking first. Have you ever had someone interrupt you? This person may have finished a sentence for you, but the thoughts were not what you wanted to say. It is important to let each person finish his or her own statement.

Your own thoughts can also distract you from listening. Poor listeners think about what they will say next rather than listening to what the other person is saying. When someone else is talking, give him or her your full attention. After the person has finished talking, you can take a few seconds to collect your thoughts if needed before responding.

Control Strong Emotions

It's good to have feelings and express those feelings. When you're listening, however, it's better to control strong emotions. Letting your emotions get out of control shows others how to "push your buttons." Some people will abuse this knowledge. You may also embarrass yourself or say something you'll regret. For this reason, keep your emotions under control even when you feel passionately about what has been said. Concentrate on what the other person is saying.

If you feel strongly about an issue, calmly express your feelings. If you feel too strongly to listen, ask to postpone the discussion until you have better control. Spend some time alone trying to determine why you feel so strongly. See Figure 9-3.

Controlling Strong Emotions: Christine's Story

Christine is a teen mom with a newborn daughter. Her mom helps quite a bit with the baby's care. Christine and her mom were discussing whether the baby should be on a feeding schedule or eat on demand. Her mom wanted to use a schedule. She had raised her children on feeding schedules. The nurse practitioner at the clinic had advised Christine to feed the baby on demand. Christine felt she should follow those instructions.

The more Christine and her mom talked about this issue, the angrier both of them became. Each thought she was right, and they weren't really getting anywhere. Christine asked her mom for a time-out from the discussion. She went to sit on the porch swing so she could think and get in touch with her feelings. Christine asked herself, "Do I feel threatened? Am I afraid of losing control? Am I afraid for the baby's health and safety? Do I resent not getting what I want?"

After thinking about it, she realized she and her mom were in a power struggle, each wanting her own way. She went back inside and calmly asked her mom to cooperate for one month. This would give her time to test and see if what the nurse practitioner suggested would work. Christine said she would switch to scheduled feedings at the end of the month if feeding on demand didn't work well. Her mom agreed. Both Christine and her mom felt good about the outcome.

9-3 In this case study, Christine provides an example for controlling strong emotions.

Use Reflecting to Show Understanding

This means you summarize the speaker's message in your own words. The purpose is to make sure the message you got is the same one the speaker meant to send. You can restate what a person has said and describe the emotions the other person expresses. Reflecting is one of the most effective ways to let people know you understand their verbal and nonverbal messages. It can also point out when what you heard is not the message the speaker meant to send. This can clarify misunderstandings.

> Valerie was very upset because she had broken up with her boyfriend. She stomped her foot and said to her mom, "Why did he have to treat me this way? Why did he have to dump me the week before the prom? What am I going to do now?" Her mom reflected, "You think it's unfair he did this to you. You're hurt and disappointed you won't have a date to the prom Friday night. You want to go but you don't want to go alone." Valerie nodded as the tears rolled down her face.

Ask Questions to Clarify

As you're listening, you may want to know more about a part of the speaker's message. This can help you understand more fully. Part of the message may be unclear to you. By asking questions, you help the speaker clarify the message. You may also ask questions to check your understanding. These questions show you're involved in the conversation and want to understand the other person.

Show Empathy

Empathy is the ability to see a situation from someone else's point of view. It means you can relate to what a person may be feeling without having those same feelings yourself. When you show empathy, you express that you can imagine what this situation must be like for him or her. You let the person know you can identify with his or her feelings. For instance, if your co-parent lost a family member, an empathetic response would be, "I'm so sorry to hear that. That must be very difficult for you. Would you like to talk about it?"

Empathy is different from sympathy. *Sympathy* means you share another person's feelings. It means when the other person is angry, you feel angry, too. Some people resent it when you say you sympathize. They don't believe you can feel exactly what they're feeling. These people would prefer for you to empathize with their situation. This respects their unique feelings and shows you care.

Give Feedback

Feedback means sharing your reaction to what was said. You can give feedback nonverbally or with verbal messages. For instance, a nod shows agreement. Laughter lets the other person know you found a joke funny. Describing how you feel about a person's message is an example of verbal feedback.

Shantell's grandmother was going to babysit for her. The baby had been fussy. Shantell explained that her teacher had suggested she play classical music for the baby when she was fussy. "You might try that if she starts to cry," Shantell said. Her grandmother responded, "That sounds like a good idea. I'll give it a try." When she heard this, Shantell nodded and smiled. She felt comfortable her wishes would be followed.

Effective Speaking

Listening is not the only valuable communication skill. You also need to learn how to speak effectively. This involves using words to convey thoughts and feelings. It helps others get to know you better. Speaking is a way to express meaning.

Finding a balance between speaking and listening is a key part of good communication. An effective speaker gets the point across, but lets the listener talk, too. As speakers, some people talk too much or too little.

When you talk too much, others soon become bored and lose interest in listening. They may also feel you're not interested in what they have to say. Taking more than your fair share of the spotlight can annoy others. Avoid being too wordy or using complicated words to share your beliefs. If talking too much is a problem for you, find another way to get attention from others.

Talking too little can also frustrate the listener. Are you the type of person who "clams up" and refuses to discuss a subject? This denies the other person the chance to hear your ideas, beliefs, and feelings. It prevents him or her from understanding you.

An effective speaker also tries to use I-messages when he or she talks. An I-message is a statement that focuses on the speaker. Most often, it begins with the word I. An example is "I felt sad when we argued because I want us to get along." An I-message works well for sharing feelings or addressing problems. On the other hand, a you-message focuses on the listener. It begins with you. An example is "You always have to argue." You-messages often blame or degrade (attack the self-esteem of) the listener. People are often angered or offended by these messages. I-messages don't have this effect. They let the listener focus on the message. For this reason, effective speakers use I-messages often.

Finally, a good speaker also chooses words his or her listeners will understand. He or she expresses beliefs, thoughts, and feelings clearly. Use the questions in Figure 9-4 to judge whether you're an effective speaker.

Evaluating Yourself as a Speaker

As a speaker, do you...
- express your thoughts clearly?
- choose words your listeners will understand?
- speak at a volume that is easily heard, but not too loud?
- talk enough but not too much?
- use I-messages?
- allow the listener to speak, too?
- control strong emotions?
- refrain from using curse words, calling names, and putting people down?
- express anger appropriately?
- communicate in an assertive, not aggressive, way?
- answer questions from your listeners to clarify your message?
- accept feedback from your listeners?
- adjust your speaking tone, style, or volume based on your listeners' feedback?

9-4 Are you an effective speaker? Use these questions to help you find out.

Learning to Handle Anger

When you're communicating with others, sometimes you will feel angry. You may be tempted to say something you know will hurt the other person. How should you handle this situation?

It is okay to feel angry. This is a normal reaction when someone has crossed your boundaries. Holding your anger inside won't help, though. Instead, it will increase your stress level. Over time, stress caused by anger can cause health problems. Dealing with your anger can help you reduce stress buildup.

The best way to release anger is to tell the other person how you feel. Often this will help the other person come back to the point of the discussion. When you deal with anger directly, this keeps it from causing an even bigger problem in your relationship. If you're upset, the other person deserves to know why. He or she can't solve the problem without first knowing what it is.

When you express anger, be sure to do it appropriately. Don't blame or degrade the other person. Don't use violence or threats to get your point across. Screaming or cursing won't help, either. Instead, talk in a calm, rational tone. Use I-messages to focus on your feelings and needs. Explain what has angered you and what you want the other person to do about it. Allow the other person to talk, too. Learning to express anger in a healthy way will improve your relationships with your child, family, and friends.

If you feel furious, it may be best to postpone the discussion. Otherwise, you may say or do things you'll later regret. Simply say, "I feel very angry right now. Let's talk about this tomorrow. That way I won't say anything I don't really mean."

If you choose to postpone the discussion, come back to it as soon as you can. Ignoring the problem won't help. The problem won't just go away. The other person deserves the chance to hear your point of view. He or she also deserves the chance to be heard. Use the time away to calm down, but then return to the discussion so the two of you can solve the problem.

Humor can also help defuse anger. If the other person says something funny, it's okay to laugh. You may also point out the humor in a situation. Often this can help both of you see things more clearly. See Figure 9-5.

Another way to keep your emotions under control might be counting slowly to yourself until you feel calm enough to continue the discussion. This might help you relax so you can express yourself without hurting the other person.

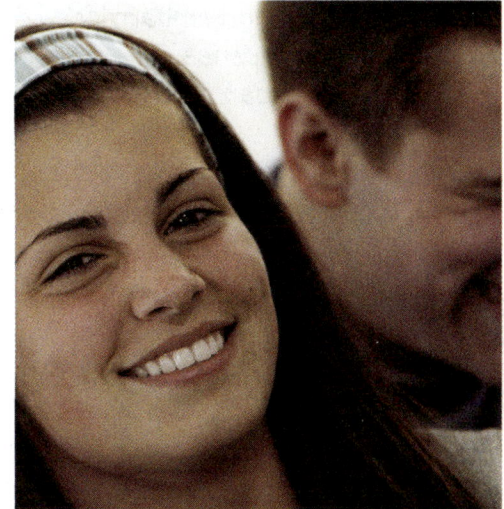

9-5 A good laugh during a heated discussion can sometimes get the conversation back on track.

Being Assertive

Dave and his girlfriend Angie were supposed to meet at the restaurant at 7:30 for their date. Dave arrived a few minutes early. He waited for Angie for over an hour. Dave was furious Angie was so late. He could handle this situation in one of three ways: by being passive, aggressive, or assertive. Which approach should Dave choose?

Passive behavior allows others to do what they want, in spite of how you feel. In this situation, Dave would have said nothing to Angie about her rude behavior. He would have pretended nothing was wrong. By responding this way, Dave's feelings and needs would have been ignored. His angry feelings wouldn't go away, though.

Aggressive behavior violates the rights of others in an attempt to get your own way. Aggression involves forceful language and rude behavior. Dave would have been aggressive if he had shouted at Angie when she arrived, "You're always late! How could you keep me waiting so long! I don't know why I even bother with you." This would have created a scene and embarrassed Angie. Dave might have felt better, but only at her expense. This message tells Angie that Dave is mad but not how she can fix the problem.

Assertive behavior allows you to express your feelings and needs directly. Dave could be assertive by talking to Angie about his feelings. After being seated at the table, he might have said quietly, "Angie, I'm disappointed you came so late. I didn't appreciate having to wait so long. Please be on time for our next date." In this approach, Dave could express his feelings while still respecting Angie. He would feel better for sharing his feelings, and Angie would know what he expected her to do. This would have been the best way to address the problem.

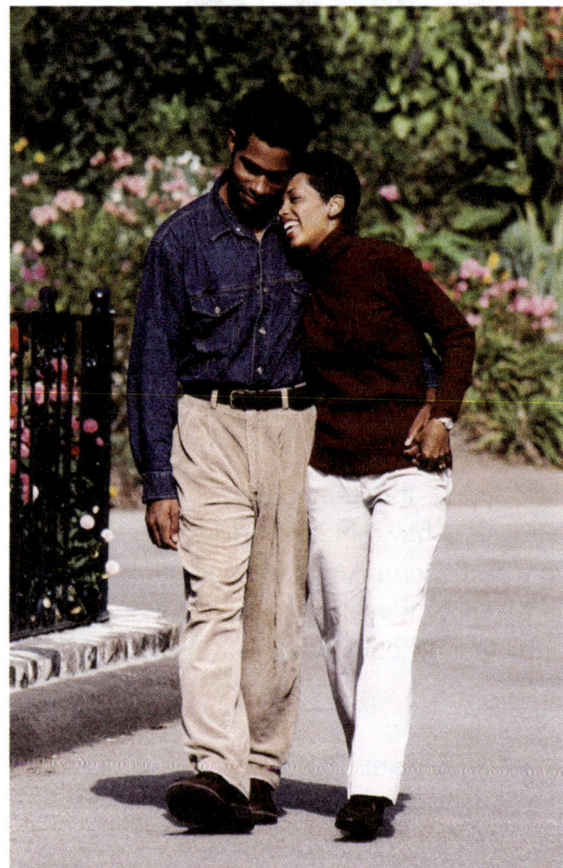

9-6 A healthy relationship is one where both partners can be assertive in expressing their feelings and needs.

In a healthy relationship, both people are assertive. See Figure 9-6. They express their feelings and needs politely but honestly. You have the right to say no when you're asked to cross your boundaries. Being assertive means standing up for your beliefs. It doesn't mean you can attack the beliefs of others. It also doesn't mean you can verbally or physically abuse others. When you're assertive, you are straightforward but show respect for others. People around you feel they have been treated fairly and honestly.

Being assertive also sets a good example for your child. By watching you, he will learn not to let others take advantage of him. He will also learn not to bully others. Your child will learn to stand up for himself. He will learn how to handle difficult situations from watching you.

Barriers to Good Communication

In spite of all your efforts to communicate clearly, you'll still have trouble at times. Try to avoid the following communication barriers:

- bringing up old issues. Stay on the subject. Discuss only the present time and situation.

- dishonesty or lack of trust. Dishonesty refers to a lack of truthfulness. Both people in a relationship need to be honest. Each person should tell the truth while still being sensitive to the other's feelings. Trust means being able to believe in and rely on someone. When trust is missing, you don't know what to believe about the speaker's message. You can't be sure your listener won't tell someone else what you've said. You're less likely to be open and honest with a listener you don't really trust.

- name-calling and cursing. Avoid calling people names or cursing at them. Do not attack a person or the person's family. These techniques make people feel they need to defend themselves. This takes the conversation away from the subject you're discussing. It can make the problem worse. Focusing on the problem at hand is a better approach.

- you-messages. For example, instead of saying, "Where were you for the last hour? You should have called," you might say, "I was really concerned when I didn't know where you were. I wish you had called me." The other person is likely to respond better to the second message than to the first. You-messages often create anger and resentment instead of solving problems. I-messages can help you express your feelings and expectations, which can lead to problem solving.

- blaming. Avoid blaming words such as <u>always</u> and <u>never</u>. Statements such as "I always have to do the laundry" are rarely completely true. They can lead to defensiveness that may create anger. Blaming often creates an atmosphere where each person accuses the other. This doesn't solve any problems.

- criticism. Be careful when offering criticism. Criticize behaviors rather than the person. Offer a possible solution rather than just stating a complaint. If you don't have a solution, ask the other person to help you find one. Make a list of possible ways to solve the issue. See Figure 9-7.

- put-downs. A *put-down* is a comment meant to make the other person look bad. The person who says it usually wants to look good. However, making the other person look bad doesn't help the speaker look any better. Put-downs also hurt the other person, which further breaks down the communication.

- prejudices. *Prejudice* is an unfair opinion or judgment made about people of another group without getting to know them. Making comments that show distrust or dislike for another group harms open communication. You may want to discuss any prejudices you have with an adult you trust. By working through these feelings, you can learn to communicate better with those around you.

- certain personality traits. Good communication can be made more difficult by some people's traits. For instance, someone who always wants the spotlight may not listen well. He or she may try to direct the discussion or do all the talking. A very shy person might speak so quietly others can't hear him or her. A person with a "know-it-all" attitude or competitive nature may make others feel what they have to say isn't valued. What other traits can you think of that might block communication?

Avoiding Criticism: John's Story

John's wife, Cora, had always been in charge of handling their bills. Lately, John felt she was managing their money poorly. He decided he would address the problems without being critical. He stated, "Cora, I've noticed we run out of money before we run out of bills. I'd like us to work together to solve this problem. I think we should think of some ways we can keep better track of the money we spend. Then we can choose the way that is most likely to work for us." Cora was glad to have help. She wasn't defensive because she had not been criticized.

9-7 In this case study, John gives Cora feedback without criticizing her.

Communicating with Others

How do you rate on the key elements of communication? What are your strongest areas, and in which ones can you stand to improve? As you evaluate yourself, set goals for improvement. You can replace your less effective communication skills with ones that will serve you better.

The communication skills you'll need depend on the person. Certain skills are best for sharing messages with your child. Others will help you and your co-parent work together. Still other skills will help you relate to your parents. Learning these skills takes practice and patience. It is well worth the effort, though. Stronger communication leads to stronger relationships.

Children

As a parent, you need to learn to communicate well with your child. This is how you will teach her about the world around her. If you work to develop good communication early, it will pave the way for better communication as she grows. The following guidelines will help you throughout your child's life:

- Remember the importance of a gentle touch. Your touch communicates your feelings for your child. A soft and tender touch makes your child feel loved and secure. See Figure 9-8. Never touch your child when you feel angry.

- Eye contact matters. Maintain eye contact with your child as you bathe and feed her. Your baby will like to listen to you talk as you look into her eyes. As a toddler, she will listen best if you get down on her level to talk with and listen to her. This allows her to look into your eyes. It

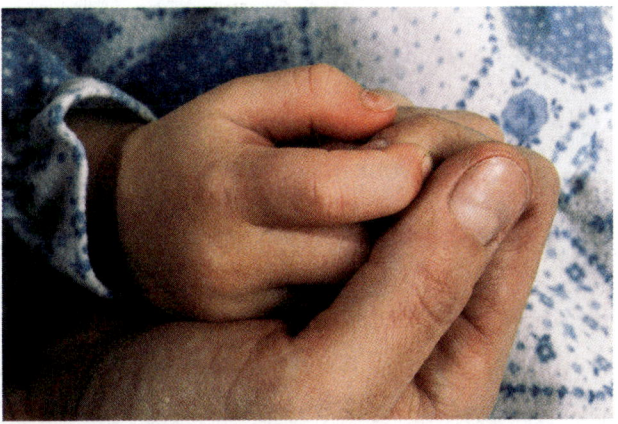

9-8 Your child enjoys a gentle touch that communicates your feelings of love and closeness.

also gets her attention if you need to explain something to her.

- ☛ Trust and honesty count. Your child needs to know she can trust you to meet her physical needs. She needs to know she can trust you with her feelings, even if it is through her cries. Being there for your child when she needs you will build a good foundation for a lasting relationship.

- ☛ Watch your tone of voice. Your child can interpret this long before she understands your words. Anger or fear in your tone may cause her to cry. A calm, soothing tone can comfort her. Save yelling for critical times, such as when your child runs toward a street with traffic. If you don't often yell, she will know to respond quickly when you do. Frequent use of yelling would only lead her to ignore it.

As your child matures, you will continue to develop new skills for communicating with her. When she is a teen, trust and honesty will be even more important. You will use the skills that are described in other sections when she is an adult.

Co-Parent

You and your child's other parent have something in common—your child. This is true whether you're married, living together, or leading separate lives. You may get along really well with your co-parent. On the other hand, it may be a struggle to even speak to him or her. Either way, you owe it to your child to communicate with this person as well as you can.

Good communication between you and your co-parent is best for your child. It means you can discuss your child's needs and how the two of you will meet them. Sharing your insights about your child's behavior can help each of you get to know him better. Talking about guidance and discipline will help you work together to parent your child.

It's also good to set and honor boundaries with your co-parent. If the two of you aren't together, you may want to set a limit stating the two of you won't talk about the past. You both may agree not to say negative things about your child in front of him. The two of you may promise not to argue or physically fight in front of your child. Boundaries create guidelines you can follow about what will be best for your child.

Part of effective communication is making time to talk regularly. You may need to ask someone to care for your child for an hour or two each week so you and your co-parent can take time to discuss matters. When your child is young, planning talks during his naps or after his bedtime may work. Keep a list of topics to discuss to help you remember what is most important.

You can also communicate with your co-parent in writing. This may help you resolve negative feelings or explain your point of view. If you're very angry, write a letter expressing yourself. In this letter, don't hold back. Use it as a way to get your thoughts together and your emotions out on paper. Don't show this letter to your co-parent, though. It could be hurtful to him or her. Tear the letter up and throw it away. Then rewrite your feelings in a more respectful way. This should be a letter your co-parent can read and understand without feeling destroyed.

It's also good to affirm your co-parent. This means expressing what you like about what he or she does. Be specific about what impresses you. For example, you could say, "The way you hold the baby must make him feel very safe." This builds your co-parent's confidence and fosters good will between you.

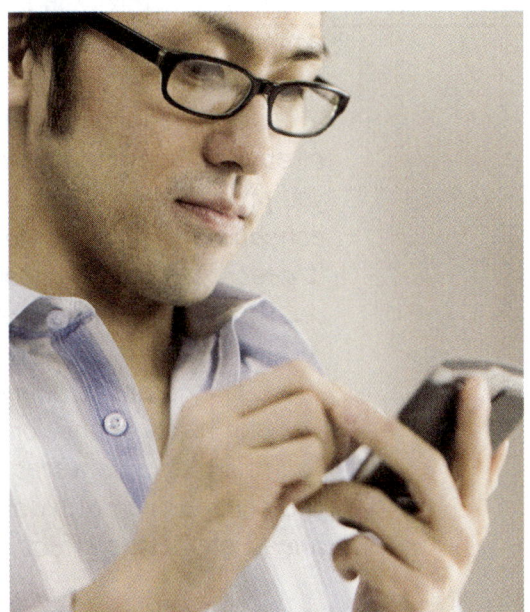

Be kind, courteous, and respectful to your co-parent. See Figure 9-9. Treating him or her in any other way sends a negative message to your child. Even if you don't like this person very much, you can still show respect for him or her. This will help you get along and parent your child as a team. When both of you use good communication skills, it also sets a good example for your child. She will learn from you how to communicate well with others.

9-9 If you and your co-parent can't always find time to meet in person, talking or sending text messages can be a good alternative.

Parents

For many families, the most stressful years are the children's teen years. Most teens want to be independent. Many parents don't think their teens are ready to be this independent. This can create conflict. When a teen is also a parent, at times it can cause even more problems in the relationship. Conflicts may arise about roles and responsibilities. For example, the teen and his or her parents may argue about the baby's other parent. They may disagree about schedules, how to parent, and other matters.

How well do you and your parents get along? Can you talk to them about what's important to you? Do you feel they understand what you're telling them? Is their message clear to you? If your relationship has been strained, you may feel like it's a lost cause. Actually, there's much you can do to help your parents understand your needs.

Communicating with your parents is very important. You may need to explain the pressures you feel. This will help them understand. Talk with them about what you see on TV and hear at school. Ask their advice on key issues.

Use I-messages when talking to your parents. For instance, instead of saying, "You're always on my back," you might say, "I feel angry when you pressure me to get off the phone to do my homework. I have set a schedule and I plan to do homework from 6:30 to 7:30." This is specific. It describes what you feel. It tells your parents why you feel the way you do. The use of I-messages builds understanding and trust.

If things aren't going well between you and your parents, perhaps you can ask a counselor or teacher for advice. This person might help you role-play a conversation with your parents. Role-playing can help you choose the right words and phrases to use. It will help you think ahead about the effect your words might have.

Communicating with others is a vital part of relationships. Do your best to communicate well with your child, co-parent, parents, and others. As you learn to communicate more effectively, you may also see an improvement in your relationships with others.

Conflict Resolution

All relationships have conflicts. You disagree with other people at times. A struggle may result, with each person wanting his or her own way. You need to know what causes disagreements and how to handle them in a healthy way. Your goal should be to reach an outcome that will help everyone involved.

Causes of Conflict

What causes these conflicts? You may argue with someone over differences of opinion. Conflicts may occur when you disagree with someone over something you value a great deal. Each of you may try to persuade the other to change his or her mind. Usually neither person wants to budge. See Figure 9-10. These conflicts can be heated.

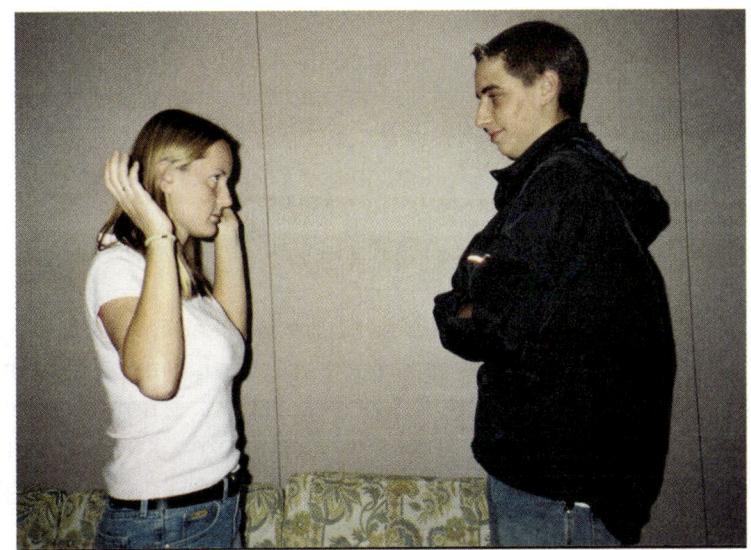

9-10 Conflicts can arise over a difference of opinion.

Some conflicts result from negative feelings. You might be angry with a friend, for instance, if you feel he or she treated you wrongly. Conflict might occur if you feel jealous of your co-parent's new partner. You might argue with your parents if you disagree with a choice they made that involves you.

You may have a personality clash with someone. This means your personality doesn't match well with the other person's. It may cause the two of you not to get along very well. A power struggle, where both people want their own way, can also lead to conflicts.

Other disputes are over trivial things. No one even remembers what started it all. Often the real cause of these conflicts is not what you're fighting over. It's often a deeper problem that needs to be resolved. Figuring out what the real problem is can help you solve these conflicts.

Each relationship is unique. What causes conflict varies from one relationship to another. This is a good point to keep in mind. As you get to know a person well, you will learn what causes conflicts between you.

Conflict Outcomes

Resolving conflicts is a big part of maintaining a relationship. How a conflict is handled will affect its outcome. Two kinds of resolution are possible. In a *constructive resolution*, everyone is satisfied with the results. It might be possible that no one person totally has his or her way. People may be angry, but they work things out. The relationship is unharmed. This is a healthy way to solve problems.

With a *destructive resolution*, feelings are hurt and negative emotions are experienced. One person may win the conflict but lose the respect of the others. Trust may be lost. Violence may occur or harsh words may be spoken. The relationship is hurt permanently. Afterward, the people involved don't respond to each other in the same way. This type of outcome is not healthy.

Ways to Handle Conflict

You can resolve a conflict in many ways. Three of these are accommodation, compromise, and collaboration. Your choice may depend on the circumstances. No one option is best for every conflict. For a few conflicts, none of these three options works.

If you choose to *accommodate*, you go along with the other person's wishes and let the person have his or her way. This can be a good choice if it doesn't clash with your values and beliefs. Going against what you believe to avoid a fight isn't a good option. Choosing someone else's way is also a poor choice if it causes you or your child to be hurt emotionally or physically. Before you choose to accommodate, be sure you can be comfortable with this option. If it leaves you with negative feelings or regrets, then it isn't the right choice.

Rosa and Hector were trying to decide which type of movie to rent. Rosa wanted to watch a romantic movie, but Hector preferred a science fiction. Hector decided nothing would be lost if he let Rosa have her way. He chose to accommodate Rosa and rent a romance. He could feel comfortable with this decision.

When conflict occurs, you may also choose *compromise*. This means each person gives a little in order to reach a middle ground. Neither of you gets all of what you wanted. Instead, each gets a little of what he or she wanted. Compromise can be a good choice when the issue isn't an ethical one. If you can accept the solution and be comfortable with it, this can be a good choice.

Keisha and Marcus were trying to choose a name for their baby, who would be born soon. Both liked Sierra for a girl's first name, but that was all the common ground they had. Marcus wanted to name a boy after himself or give a girl his mother's name as a middle name. Keisha wanted to name a boy Joshua Tyvon and give a daughter her name as a middle name. After much discussion, Keisha and Marcus reached a compromise. They agreed Marcus could name a son, but Keisha would name a daughter. Both felt they could accept this option.

A third option is *collaboration*. This is when everyone involved works together to find a solution that is acceptable to all. It is a win-win situation. Everyone feels good about the decision. In collaboration, all participants are a part of the solution. See Figure 9-11.

Steps in Conflict Resolution

When you're involved in a conflict, the goal is to reach a constructive outcome. To do this, everyone must work together to solve the problem. If the conflict is heated, you may need to ask someone who is not involved to lead the discussion. This person

> **Collaboration: Tia's Story**
>
> Tia is a teen mom. She and her parents hadn't been getting along well. They kept saying she was spending too much time with her boyfriend and not enough with her baby and her homework. Tia was upset because she felt they were nagging her.
>
> Tia asked for a family meeting to discuss these issues. In the meeting, her parents shared their fears and their hopes for her future. They explained how caring for her baby so often was limiting their time as a couple. Tia described her dreams and goals. She shared how much she valued her relationships with them, her baby, and her boyfriend. Tia reassured her parents her education meant as much to her as it did to them.
>
> Tia and her parents decided to work together to reach an agreement that would meet everyone's needs. They created a chart on which Tia could track time spent with her baby, her boyfriend, and her studies. The chart also tracked time watching TV, sleeping, and doing other activities. After a week, the trends were obvious. Tia was spending more time with her boyfriend than she realized. She was also spending less time with the baby and her homework than she had thought.
>
> Tia asked her parents to help her budget her time. They worked together to create a schedule. It included time with her boyfriend, as well as plenty of time for the baby and her studies. The schedule worked well, and everyone was happy with the results. They agreed that collaboration worked well in this situation.

9-11 In this case study, Tia and her parents collaborate to solve a problem.

wouldn't give an opinion or choose the solution. He or she would only help the group talk to one another and stay focused. To resolve a conflict, try using the following six steps:

- Identify the problem. Everyone must agree on what the problem is. Sometimes this is more complicated than it sounds. Completing this step will clarify the issue. It will give you some guidance in finding the solution.

- Brainstorm possible solutions. When brainstorming, don't judge or criticize others or their thoughts. List all ideas and possible solutions. Often the best suggestions come after people think they've run out of ideas.

- Evaluate the possible solutions. Work together to create a set of questions to ask about each option. These can include questions about practicality and results. Set other criteria for the solution. Find out who would agree to each option. Modify any solutions that don't meet the criteria. If an option doesn't meet the criteria and can't be revised, cross

Chapter 9   Communicating for Better Relationships

it off the list. Also change or throw out any options that can't be agreed to by all.

- Choose the best solution. Everyone must agree to it or the conflict isn't resolved. Evaluate the solution. Is it working? Is anyone still unhappy with the solution and results? If so, go through the steps again. If you didn't have someone mediate the first time, it may be wise to do so now. You may also seek help from a counselor or other professional.

- Accept the results. If it becomes necessary, agree to disagree. Work together to prevent flare-ups of anger over the issue. Accept the results of your chosen solution. Put the dispute behind you and focus on the relationship instead.

How you handle conflict will have a lasting effect on your relationships. Learning to handle it in a mature way will help you be happier. It will also model for your child how to handle conflicts as she matures.

Major Points

- Communication, or the exchanging of messages, is a vital part of relationships. It helps you share your thoughts, feelings, and experiences with others. It can help you get to know others and learn about the world around you.

- You can use both verbal and nonverbal communication to send and receive messages. While verbal messages use words, nonverbal messages rely on more subtle cues such as body language and tone of voice.

- Listening is a key part of communication. This skill is different from hearing, in that it includes understanding what has been said. Active listening skills can help you better understand the messages being sent.

- Effective speaking is important, too. It helps others understand what you have to say. By learning to be a good speaker, you can improve your relationships with others.

- While it's healthy to feel anger, it can damage your relationship if you express it in the wrong way. Learn to share your feelings with others in a respectful way that helps them understand. Being assertive with others is also important.

- Many habits and communication styles are barriers to good communication. They can get in the way of sending and receiving clear messages. To improve your communication skills, learn to avoid these barriers.

- You can use special communication skills when talking with your child, co-parent, and parents. Use these techniques in addition to basic communication skills. As you gain practice, you may notice your relationships improve.

- Conflicts occur in all relationships from time to time. They can have many causes and can vary in intensity. By learning to handle and resolve conflict, you can work out your differences with others. This can allow you to maintain key relationships despite conflict.

Chapter 10
Crises in Relationships

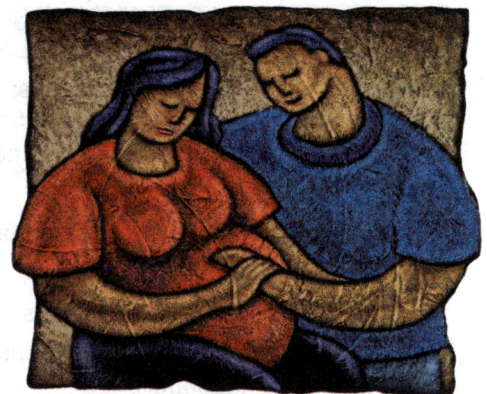

A *crisis* is a situation that causes distress and interrupts a person's normal way of thinking and coping. It is a situation that cannot be escaped but demands change and adjustment. During a crisis, a person's normal coping skills won't work. The person must adapt and find new coping skills. Crises also cause intense emotions, often negative ones, that a person must work through. These tasks take time and effort to accomplish.

Everyone will experience some crises in life. That doesn't mean it's easy, though. Some crises surround positive changes. Others are the result of bad things that have happened. See Figure 10-1 for some examples of crises.

Whether a situation is a crisis depends on the person. What is experienced as a crisis for one person might not be a crisis for someone else. If you can use your normal coping skills to easily adjust to a situation, it is not a crisis for you. If you must develop new coping skills to deal with this problem, this may be a crisis. It will take you time to adjust and make the changes needed. How much you are affected emotionally by the situation may also tell you whether it's a crisis.

In this chapter, you will learn about some common crises teens face. It's possible you or someone you know might face one or more of these crises. Learning about them may help you prevent them or lessen their effect. You will also learn about how people respond to crisis and what types of help are available.

What Is a Crisis?

Many situations or events can present themselves as crises. Some are positive changes, while others are not. Keep in mind that what is a crisis for one person might not be for someone else. The following are some events that might cause crises among families:

- birth or adoption of a baby
- relative moving into or out of the family home
- marriage or remarriage
- divorce or separation of spouses
- death (or suicide) of a family member
- unexpected pregnancy
- miscarriage or stillbirth of a baby
- long-term hospitalization or nursing home care of a family member
- addictions
- family member committing or being accused of a crime
- having a child or teen run away from home
- having a spouse desert the family
- loss of a job
- bankruptcy
- poverty, homelessness, or starvation
- depression
- disability of a family member
- natural disasters, such as tornadoes, floods, hurricanes, earthquakes, or fires
- being the victim of a crime (theft, robbery, rape, homicide, shooting, assault, vandalism)
- breakup of a romantic relationship or close friendship
- war or rioting
- abuse, neglect, or incest
- poor health, serious illness, or disability of a family member
- serious accident or injury

10-1 Many situations can create a crisis. What other examples can you identify?

Common Crises for Teens

You will face some personal crises in your life. Your family will encounter crises from time to time. A crisis might occur within a relationship, too. Crises can affect the way you interact with others. You may draw closer to loved ones or pull away. Not everyone responds in the same way. Each person and each crisis is unique.

Some crises are more common than others among teens. These are depression, domestic violence, sexual assault, rape, incest, and addictions. By learning more about these crises, perhaps you can recognize them if they occur in your life or happen to someone you know.

Depression

Feeling down sometimes is normal. Everyone deals with disappointments and problems. Sometimes these can lead you to feel sad or upset. If you feel this way all or most of the time, however, you may have *depression*. If so, you're likely to be overwhelmed by intense feelings of sadness and hopelessness. You may not even know why you feel this way. If you do know why, you may not know what to do about it. This is a common but scary problem to have.

You may wonder how to know if you're depressed. Many signs can indicate you have this problem. See Figure 10-2. If you have five or more of these signs, you may be severely depressed. This can interfere with your ability to function normally and be happy. You need to seek help immediately so you can resolve this problem.

Signs of Depression

Common signs of depression include the following:
- depressed mood most of the day, nearly every day
- loss of interest or pleasure in favorite activities
- change in appetite without dieting—weight loss or weight gain
- change in sleeping patterns—trouble sleeping or sleeping too much
- change in activity level—restlessness, agitation, or inactivity
- constant tiredness, fatigue, or loss of energy
- feelings of worthlessness or excessive guilt
- difficulty thinking or concentrating
- being overwhelmed with thoughts of the problem
- greater indecisiveness than usual
- frequent thoughts of death or suicide

10-2 When a person is depressed, he or she will show some of these warning signs.

Depression can have many causes. It may be a response to other crises occurring in your life. For instance, if you lose your job or break up with your partner, you might feel down about this. Severe depression can also be a crisis of its own, however. It can last a long time and require professional help to resolve. Learning the signs of depression can help you identify it if it happens to you. Finding a way to cope with depression is important. This will allow you to recover and find happiness again.

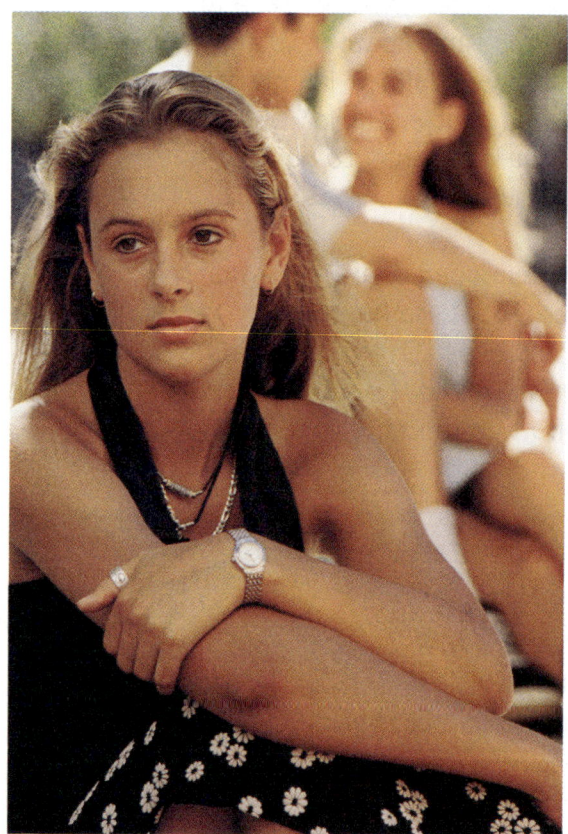

10-3 In pregnant teens and teen moms, depression may be a result of hormonal changes.

An imbalance of certain chemicals in the brain can cause depression. This type of depression can be treated with medication. The medicine corrects the balance of the chemicals in the brain, which lifts the person's mood.

For women, other physical changes in the body can trigger depression. This is most true for pregnant women and new mothers. As a woman's body adjusts first to being pregnant and then to not being pregnant anymore, her hormone levels will change. These major changes can affect mood and blood sugar levels. This can cause an imbalance in her system that may result in depression. See Figure 10-3. For most women, these depressed feelings last only a short time. They are called baby blues. Some women experience more extreme and lasting feelings of depression. This is known as postpartum depression. A woman should talk to her health care provider if she suspects she might have this type of depression.

Taking poor care of yourself can also cause depression. To feel your best, you need to eat well, be active, and rest enough. Avoiding harmful substances, such as drugs and alcohol is important, too. Following these good health habits shows you care about yourself and what happens to you. Failing to take care of yourself can lead to depression. Guilt over poor health habits can make matters even worse.

Feeling that a situation is hopeless may also cause depression. Facing many failures or disappointments in a short period of time can also bring people down. Negative thoughts have a big effect on a person's mood. For example, self-pity, or feeling sorry for oneself, can also lead to depression. A person may think, "Nothing ever goes my way." This belief can keep a person from trying, and make the situation even worse.

Most people feel depressed at one time or another. Many times, this feeling soon passes. A mild bout of depression that is short-lived may not be a crisis. It may just be a down time in your life that you quickly get over. You can overcome a mild case of depression by using your personal resources. If you eat better, rest, and exercise, your mood may really improve. Talking with friends or loved ones may ease your negative feelings. Relaxing and doing activities you enjoy will help. Soon you will feel better again.

When depression is severe, however, it can become a crisis. This is true if the feelings of depression are disabling or if they persist. If depression keeps you from being able to function, it can be a serious problem. You will likely need some help to overcome your depressed mood. Talk to a parent, caseworker, health care provider, teacher, or other trusted adult. Ask this person to assist you in finding professional help. Working with a counselor can help you resolve your feelings of hopelessness. This will ease your depression and help you function again.

Suicide

When a person is severely depressed, he or she may think of suicide. This is the act of taking one's own life. The person may be overwhelmed by problems and see no other way out of them. Life may seem so bad to him or her that death seems like a way to escape.

A person who is considering suicide may say life doesn't seem worth living. He or she may talk about giving up or ending it all. These statements are actually pleas for help. Giving away valued possessions can be another warning sign.

If someone you know is severely depressed or shows any of these signs, talk to him or her about it. Take the situation seriously. Find out how the person feels and why. Ask directly if the person is considering suicide. If so, let him or her know how much you don't want this to happen. The person will likely be relieved to know you care so much. Remind the person that death is a final step with painful consequences for friends and family. When the person considers the finality of death, he or she may see how many reasons there are to live. This can give the person the motivation he or she needs.

If you can, stay with the person and seek help at once. If it's an emergency, call a suicide hot line or the police department immediately. These trained professionals can assist you and your loved one through this crisis. Until help arrives, you can follow the tips in Figure 10-4.

Tips for Talking to a Suicidal Person

- Offer emotional support and let the person express his or her feelings.
- Treat the person with respect; never deny the feelings expressed or imply the person shouldn't feel that way.
- Assist the person in exploring other options and identifying what might help.
- Avoid arguing, challenging the person, or trying to shock him or her into reality.
- Reassure the person these feelings are temporary and will pass in time.
- Help the person identify reasons for living.
- Mention that death is final and can never be reversed.
- Remind the person of loved ones who would be affected by the suicide.
- Do not leave the person alone if depression is severe; create a physically and emotionally safe environment for him or her.

If someone you know is planning suicide, call for help. Stay with the person and keep talking until help arrives. Use these tips in your conversation.

Even if it seems the person is in no immediate danger, you have a duty to let someone know what he or she said. Your loved one is a danger to himself or herself. This person needs help. The only way to get this help is tell someone who can help. This would be a responsible adult or the police. Your loved one might be mad at you for doing this, but it could save his or her life. On the other hand, seeking help might be just what your loved one wants you to do. You would feel terrible if you kept this secret and your loved one committed suicide. By telling someone who can help, you're doing all you can to help.

Domestic Violence

A crisis faced by some teens and their families is domestic violence. This is any action meant to hurt a family member or dating partner. The abuser is the person who hurts one or more loved ones. The victim is the person being hurt. Domestic violence often, but not always, occurs among people who live in the same house. It happens most often in the following relationships:

- dating partners or spouses
- an adult relative (often a parent) and a child
- an adult relative (often the son or daughter) and an elderly person

As you might imagine, domestic violence is a crisis because of the hurt it causes. It can also damage the relationship between the abuser and the victim. A healthy relationship is one based on respect and equality. In an abusive relationship, the abuser feels he or she must have the power and control at all cost. Neither partner can trust the other. This type of relationship is not healthy for either person.

Abuse can also affect the relationships each person has with others. Both people may pull away from friends and family as they try to hide the abuse. The abuser doesn't want to get into trouble for his or her actions. For this reason, he or she threatens the victim with more abuse if anyone finds out. Out of fear and embarrassment, the victim keeps the abuse a secret, too. Isolating themselves from loved ones makes it more difficult for them to seek help and end the abuse.

Why would someone hurt a family member? No one explanation exists. The reasons are complex. Most often, domestic violence is an abuser's way to feel powerful and control others. The abuser intimidates loved ones into following his or her wishes. When a family member defies these wishes, the abuser will use violence to punish him or her.

Who would treat their family members in this way? This question also has no simple answers. There is no easy way to spot an abuser. A majority of abusers are male, but some are women. Abusers can be young or old, poor or rich, and uneducated or highly educated. They come from all ethnic and religious groups.

You can't tell an abuser by looking at him or her. There are some traits common among most abusers, though. Abusers are usually unhappy people with a lot of anger. They may have problems at work or be unemployed. They may not feel a part of the family or community. Abusers have not learned to control their emotions, especially their anger. They may be impulsive (act without first thinking about the consequences). Abusers feel out of control over some aspect of their lives. They abuse family members to prove they have control over them.

An abuser may have unrealistic expectations of others. He or she might expect them to do things they aren't capable of doing. For example, a one-year-old cannot be expected to use the toilet. An elderly person may not be able to remember to take his or her medicine. A violent incident could occur when the victim doesn't meet the abuser's unrealistic expectations.

Many abusers were abused as children. They have learned this behavior in their families. These abusers may not see their behavior as wrong. Instead, they may think it is normal. They may not know other ways to interact with people or express their feelings.

High levels of stress may lead a person to abuse loved ones. This is often the case for parents who commit child abuse. The abuser may feel overwhelmed by problems and unable to cope. He or she might take this out on others, such as the children. Sometimes this abuse is caused by parents who are unhappy in their parenting role or feel unprepared to meet their children's needs.

Many abusers also have problems with alcohol or drugs. Using these substances can lower their ability to think clearly and act appropriately. They may be more likely to abuse others when they use these substances.

Abuse can occur for other reasons, too. These can vary according to the family in which the abuse takes place. Each case is unique.

Who is to blame for the abuse? The abuser is always responsible for his or her actions. He or she chooses to use abusive behavior against others. This is wrong. There may be factors, such as stress or substance abuse, that make the abuse more likely. These factors can explain the abuse, but they do not excuse it. No matter what example is set for a person, he or she must decide whether to follow it.

Some victims blame themselves for the abuse. They think their actions caused the other person to hurt them. They may feel they deserved the abuse. Abusers commonly try to make their victims feel this way. They may say, "You made me hit you. You should have done as I told you." In reality, no matter what a victim says or does, he or she did not cause the abuse. Every person is responsible for his or her own actions. The abuser, not his or her family or victims, is to blame for the abuse. An abuser chooses whether to hurt others or treat them with respect.

Forms of Abuse

You may wonder which behaviors are abusive. Each state has an exact legal definition of abuse. These can vary from state to state. The law is always most clear about child abuse, or abuse occurring to a person younger than 18 years old. It is also most exact about physical abuse. This describes injuries someone purposely causes to a person's body. See Figure 10-5.

Examples of Physical Abuse	
• hitting	• whipping
• kicking	• stalking
• slapping	• throwing things
• punching	• using objects to beat a person
• biting	• using hot substances to burn a person
• pushing	• using or threatening to use weapons to hurt a person
• grabbing	
• restraining	• preventing a person from leaving the house

10-5 This list gives examples of physical abuse. Can you think of others?

Other forms of abuse are harder to measure and detect. That doesn't make them any less painful or any less wrong, however. These include emotional abuse, sexual abuse, and neglect.

Emotional abuse is behavior that hurts feelings or damages self-esteem. This includes name-calling, degrading, and **belittling** (to cause someone to seem or feel less of a person). The abuser may make the victim feel worthless, unloved, and less of a person. An abuser may tell the victim no one else will ever love him or her. Playing mind games and trying to make the victim feel crazy are emotional abuse, too. Abusers often accuse their spouses or partners of cheating on them. For this reason, an abuser might control the victim's use of the car, mail, telephone, or computer.

Sexual abuse means abuse involving sexual activity or issues. This might or might not include forced intercourse, which is called **rape**. Forcing a person to view or participate in sexual acts or materials is sexual abuse. The type of sexual abuse most commonly reported involves children who are abused by adults. Sexual abuse can also happen between dating partners or spouses. This often goes unreported, though. Victims may not know being forced into sex by a dating partner or spouse is wrong. They may also fear no one will believe them.

Neglect means holding back or failing to provide things that are needed. An example is failing to provide food, clothing, or medical care. When parents don't give their child the supervision he needs, this is neglect. Leaving a young child at home alone is also illegal. Failing to provide the physical care a child needs is also neglect. Neglect can also be keeping a child out of school or not making sure he gets to school each day. Failing to provide a child with a coat in the winter is a sign of neglect. Emotional neglect can be withholding love, praise, or attention from a child.

An elderly person might also be a victim of neglect. A caretaker may fail to provide the needed food or medicine. The abuser may refuse to help the person turn over, get in and out of bed, and use the toilet. He or she may not keep the elderly person's body, clothes, and bedding clean. The abuser might withhold devices the person needs to function. These might include glasses, hearing aids, canes, and walkers. All these actions are neglect.

Seeking Help

No matter what its form, domestic violence is a crisis. It endangers the victim's emotional and physical well-being. Abuse can take away a person's self-esteem and threaten his or her safety. It can destroy relationships and families. In severe cases, domestic violence can result in death. Even in less severe cases, it can leave painful and lasting emotional and physical scars.

Some people think domestic violence is a family problem and shouldn't be reported to the police. Others think it is important to report it so the family can get help. This can give them hope of a better future. Every state has laws against abuse. The police can intervene in cases of abuse. Abusers can be fined, ordered to get counseling, or sent to jail.

A victim can also ask the court to grant an order of protection. This court order sets clear terms to protect a victim from abuse. It sets limits on the contact the abuser can have with the victim. While it is in force, an order of protection can also set terms for the possession of a shared home and the custody and support of children. (To learn more about orders of protection, see another title in this series, Building Your Future.)

When child abuse occurs, it should be reported to the police or the department of child and family services. This allows the abuse to be investigated and possibly result in the abuser's arrest. In many states, certain professionals are mandated reporters of child abuse. This means they are required by law to report any known or suspected cases of child abuse. Health care providers, counselors, child care workers, and teachers are often mandated reporters. See Figure 10-6. Anyone can

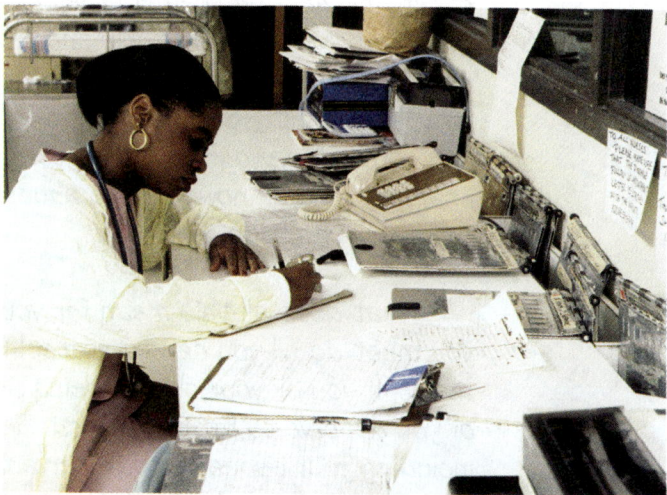

10-6 This nurse is bound by law to report any child abuse she knows about or suspects. She is a mandated reporter of child abuse.

report child abuse, though. If you know or strongly suspect a child is being abused, you should call to report it. Give all the information you have so the case can be investigated. This is often the only way child abuse can be ended. It can be the first step to getting the child and the abuser the help they need.

In partner abuse, unless something interrupts the pattern of abuse, it will continue. Since the abuser doesn't see his or her actions as wrong, it is usually the victim who must seek help first. Often this means leaving the violent relationship.

To get away safely, victims can often escape to shelters for battered women and their children. Many communities have these shelters. They provide safe short-term emergency housing for victims of abuse. These programs also provide emotional support, counseling, food, clothing, and personal items. They may also offer job training and help in finding a new place to live. Victims can ask health care providers, counselors, police officers, or religious leaders how to find these shelters. Most shelters run domestic violence hot lines. Victims can call these hot lines for advice, support, or information. They can also call to request shelter.

Abusers need help, too. Many counseling programs can help abusers learn to deal better with their anger and stop hurting others. By getting the help they need, abusers can feel more control over their lives. This can help them stop their abusive actions. Most often, abusers enter these programs because they are ordered to do so by the court. Abusers can seek this help on their own, too. They can contact a program for batterers or seek individual counseling. For change to occur, however, the abuser must sincerely want to stop his or her hurtful behavior.

What does all this mean for you and your relationships? First, you must do all you can to protect yourself and your child from abuse. If you or your child is being abused, seek help at once. Neither of you deserve to be mistreated. Second, you must not abuse others, including your spouse or partner and your child. See Figure 10-7. Be honest with yourself about whether your words or actions are abusive to others. If so, you must seek help to stop this hurtful behavior.

Taking Steps to Prevent Abuse

As an Abuser	As a Victim
Find someone to talk to about your negative feelings.	Watch for warning signs of a potential abuser. Avoid becoming more involved with someone you suspect might be an abuser.
Learn to form more realistic expectations of others.	Avoid spending all your time with your partner and neglecting other important relationships.
Work to build your self-esteem without degrading others.	Become assertive rather than passive.
Ask for help with your child if you feel very angry.	Set clear limits and stick to them. Make it clear you will not accept abuse or mistreatment from anyone.
Learn to take a time-out from situations when you're enraged.	Be willing to leave a bad relationship. Avoid settling for a poor relationship over being alone.
Seek support from loved ones.	Realize you cannot change a person and abusive behavior usually only gets worse over time.
Work with community agencies to gain more control over other areas of your life.	Report abuse to the authorities every time it occurs.
Avoid drugs and alcohol.	Seek counseling.
Learn what your triggers are and work on them.	Put your safety and your children's safety first at all times.
Work to communicate more clearly.	Be cautious when entering a new relationship. Take your time getting to know the person.
Become assertive rather than aggressive.	Avoid relationships in which you're expected to give up your own identity, power, or control.
Seek counseling.	Set goals and pursue activities that make you feel complete as a person. Avoid defining yourself in terms of your relationship.
Make a commitment not to abuse or control others.	Work to build your self-esteem. Learn to accept yourself and love who you are. Avoid counting on a relationship
Attend an anger management class.	Learn to communicate more effectively.

10-7 Follow these tips to lower your chances of abusing others or being abused.

Seeking help to end abuse is the only way to save the relationship. An abusive relationship is unhealthy and unsatisfying for everyone involved. By finding help right away, the chance remains that the relationship can be rebuilt. For this to happen, however, both people must be committed to having a healthy relationship. They will have to learn new ways to interact with one another. This will take time, effort, and help, but it can be done.

Sexual Assault, Rape, and Incest

Another type of crisis is being the victim of a sexual crime. This crisis is serious and can have lasting emotional effects. The victim feels violated and unable to trust others. The trauma of a sexual crime can be difficult to overcome. Healing may take a long time and require professional counseling.

With some sexual crimes, the perpetrator (person committing the crime) may be a stranger. Being attacked by a stranger and forced to engage in sexual behavior is traumatic. It may take years for the victim to feel safe again.

In many cases, though, the perpetrators of sexual crimes are known to the victims. They may be acquaintances or loved ones. Being forced into unwanted sexual behavior by a dating partner, spouse, or relative can be devastating. Along with feeling violated, the victim feels betrayed by someone close to her.

One sexual crime is sexual assault. This refers to any kind of forced sexual behavior. In sexual assault, the perpetrator may be a stranger or someone the victim knows. Sexual assault includes unwanted touching and forced or coerced sexual behavior. This crime can result in jail time.

Rape is one specific type of sexual assault. Rape occurs when a person is forced to have intercourse against his or her wishes. In many states, the legal definition of rape includes vaginal, oral, and anal intercourse. There can be one or more perpetrators. The law allows strict criminal sentences for rapists.

Chapter 10   Crises in Relationships

Date rape is rape that occurs between people who are dating or dated in the past. In this crime, one partner forces the other to have sex. Under the law, this type of rape is every bit as wrong as rape by a stranger.

Marital rape is forced sex that occurs between spouses. In the past, this type of rape wasn't always considered a crime. However, now all but a few states have made marital rape illegal. Just because spouses can and do have a sexual relationship does not give either partner the right to force the other into unwanted sexual activity.

You can take precautions to help prevent sexual assault, including rape. Most assaults are spontaneous rather than planned. Sexual assault can occur anywhere and at any time. Dark and secluded areas carry a higher risk for stranger rape. However, rape can even occur in public areas such as parks and shopping malls during the daylight. Many sexual assaults take place in the home or car of the victim or perpetrator. It's important to have a plan for protecting yourself from sexual assault. Consider the tips in Figure 10-8 as you make your plan.

After a rape, the victim should go to the nearest emergency room at once. See Figure 10-9. The victim should not shower, wash, douche, change clothes, or use the bathroom. Any of these actions could destroy needed evidence. This evidence will be collected at the hospital during a medical exam. This evidence can be used to prosecute the rapist. The health care provider will treat any injuries that resulted from the rape. Tests can be done to show whether a pregnancy or STI was present before the rape occurred. Testing again a few weeks or months later can reveal whether the rape caused an STI or pregnancy.

At the hospital, the victim can give a report to police about the incident. Talking about what has happened can be traumatic, but it's important. By sharing all the details, the victim can give the police enough information to help them catch the rapist. This is the only way to punish the rapist and reduce the chance the rapist will do the same thing to someone else.

Precautions Against Sexual Assault and Rape

By Strangers

At Home

- Keep doors and windows locked at all times. Whether you are at home or away, this is a good rule to follow.
- Ask persons at the door to identify themselves. Do not open the door to strangers or people you don't trust. Ask repair and service people for ID. Use a chain guard or a peephole to see the person's ID before letting him or her in. When in doubt, ask the person to leave and call the police if he or she won't leave.
- Do not leave notes on the door telling where you are or when you will be back. This can tell an assailant exactly what to plan or expect.
- Do not go into your home alone if you feel someone has been in it or the door is open when you return. Surprising an intruder is dangerous. Call the police and have them go through your house first.
- Never leave a key in an obvious place. If you must leave a key outside, put it in a very unlikely place.
- Keep your entry well lit.
- When you approach your home, have your keys ready and go inside quickly.
- Use the buddy system at night. Go and come with another person whenever possible.
- If you are alone, call friends or family to let them know you've gotten home safely.

In Automobiles

- Park your car in a lighted area. This will allow you to see the area around your car as you return to it.
- As you approach your car, always have your keys ready. Before you reach your car, look under it, around it, and in the backseat to be sure no one is waiting for you. Enter the car as soon as possible and lock the door.
- Keep your car in good repair and full of gas. If you must call for help, call a reliable service station or insurance program. Do not accept help from strangers.
- If your car stalls, get out quickly, open the hood, and turn on the flashing hazard lights. Get back into your car and lock the door. When someone stops to help, ask them to call the police. Stay in your locked car. If a police officer stops, he or she will show you identification. If not, do not open your door.
- If you believe someone is following you, drive directly to a police station or to a place with lots of people. Do not drive to your home.
- Never leave your house keys on the key chain with your car keys at service stations, valet stands, or car washes. These could be easily copied and used later to enter your home.

(continued)

10-8 Taking precautions can help you protect yourself against sexual assault, whether by strangers or by dates.

Precautions Against Sexual Assault and Rape

By Dates

- Be cautious on first dates. Group dates offer less private time, so they're usually safer. If the two of you go out alone, choose public activities with a lot of people around. Set a definite time to be home and tell your parents where you're going and when to expect you home.
- Avoid drugs and alcohol. Most date rapes occur when these substances are used during the date. While these substances cloud a person's thinking, they are not an excuse for the rapist.
- Respect the limits your parents have set for you. Follow their rules about curfew, activities, and dating partners.
- Use good judgment in your behavior. Communicate clearly if you don't want or expect to have sex. Excessive flirting or sexual teasing may lead the other person to think you want to have sex. (This doesn't cause or excuse rape, however. It is still the other person's responsibility to make sure you consent to any sexual activity before proceeding. No <u>always</u> means no.)
- Avoid dating someone who is much older than you. Often, this person may be more likely than someone your own age to expect sex. This expectation may lead your date to force sex.
- Avoid pressures or requests to go to a more private place "to talk" or "to get to know each other." Your date may think that by saying this he or she is inviting you to have sex.
- Take enough money with you on dates to be able to call for a ride home or take a bus, train, or cab, if needed.
- Trust your instincts. End a date early or avoid further dates with someone who makes you feel uncomfortable or tries to make you feel bad for saying no.
- If you feel you're in danger, make a scene. You may fear this would embarrass you. Instead, it may alert someone to help you or buy you time to get away.

(continued)

Incest is another type of sexual crime. It is defined as sexual activity that occurs between family members other than spouses. Incest is against the law. Often, incest involves sexual activity between a parent and a child. It can involve other types of relatives, however. Incest usually involves keeping secrets from the rest of the family. This can lead to a lack of trust that damages relationships within the family.

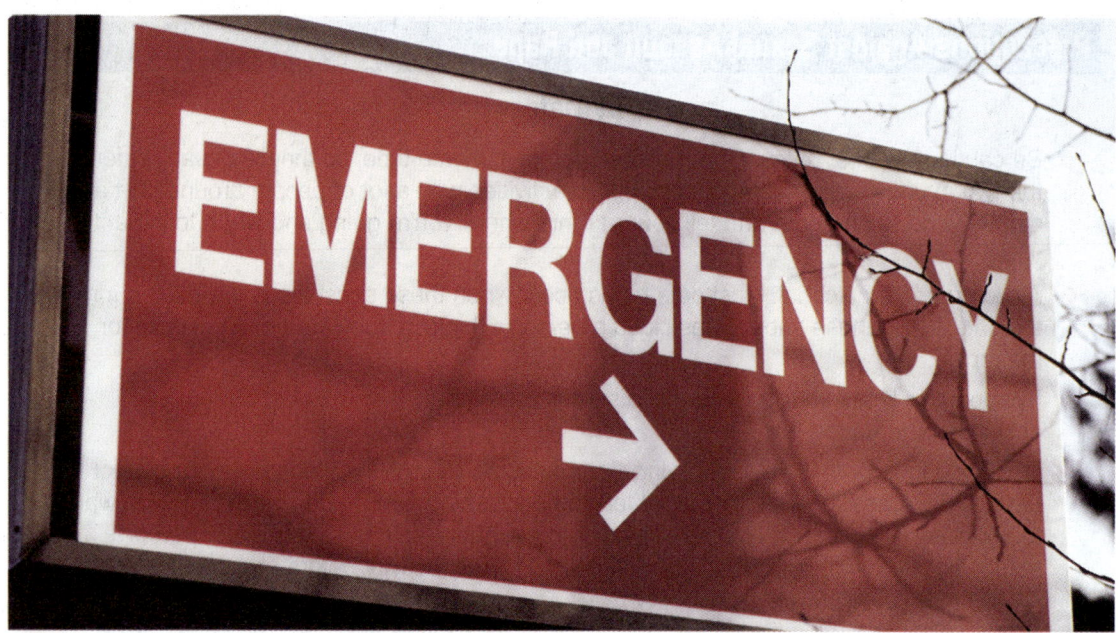

10-9 If rape occurs, it is important for the victim to go to the emergency room right away.

Most often, incest is not a single event but behavior that continues over time. Many times, incest will last for years before it is discovered or revealed. This is most often true of cases involving young children. A child may not know that what's happening is wrong. The child loves and trusts the perpetrator. This person may use bribes, tricks, or threats, to get his or her way. In the beginning, it may include only slight touching. Over time, as incidents grow more frequent and severe, the child may start to question the relationship. The child may also sense something is wrong as he or she matures and begins to understand what's happening.

Even when the victim knows what's going on, telling someone can be difficult. The victim may be afraid to report the incest. The perpetrator may have made threats to him or her. The victim may worry that an arrest would break up the family and take away from the family income. Despite these concerns, it is still important for the victim to seek help.

If you have been the victim of a sexual crime, know that what happened was not your fault. Nothing you did or failed to do caused the other person's behavior. You did not deserve to have this happen to you, and you were powerless to stop it.

The good news is you're a survivor. You can find help in overcoming this crisis. Start by talking to a parent, health care provider, religious leader, or other trusted adult. Find out if there is a sexual assault crisis center in your area. If so, you can find counseling through this agency. The crisis center might even offer free support groups. In these groups, members can support each other because they've had similar experiences. These groups are usually led by a counselor or therapist. Attending a support group or counseling might be a good idea.

Substance Abuse and Addiction

Alcohol, tobacco, and other drugs alter the way a person's mind and body function. People sometimes use these substances in an effort to relax or deal with stress. When the use of these substances interferes with a person's life, this is known as substance abuse. The drug or its effects might affect a person's job and family responsibilities.

One step further than substance abuse is addiction. An addiction to a drug means the person's body or mind has begun to depend on it. The person can't function without it. When a person is addicted to alcohol, tobacco, or other drugs, this is considered a crisis because of the way it affects his or her life. The drug alters the person's mind and body. The addiction can damage a person's health, reputation, and career.

Addiction is a crisis in relationships, too. Using the drug becomes more important than everything else, including loved ones. A person might jeopardize the well-being of friends or family. He or she might lie, steal, and commit crimes to continue this habit. The addict may spend all the family's money. Friends and family may feel they are losing the addict to his or her addiction. The person they once knew seems to be gone. It's painful for them to watch their loved one damaging himself or herself and others. Friends and family feel powerless to stop the person from using the drug. They may blame themselves or wish there was more they could do.

Most people with addictions don't want to admit they have them. Neither do their families. For this reason, it can sometimes take years for an addict to admit and deal with this problem. An addict may feel shame and fear. Often the situation must get to an all-time low before action is taken to begin the long journey toward better personal and family health.

When an addict tries to stop using the drug, he or she will feel certain symptoms. This is known as withdrawal. An addict will feel these symptoms as his or her body rids itself of the drug. Common withdrawal symptoms are irritability, nervousness, nausea, vomiting, shaking, cramps, and sleeplessness. When the drug is out of the person's system, the symptoms will go away. Going through withdrawal is very uncomfortable. If a person needs help, he or she can check into a drug rehabilitation center. These centers provide treatment, supervision, and support that help a person through withdrawal. They also offer counseling and support groups for recovering addicts.

Many self-help groups are also available at no cost to people recovering from addictions. Two of the most common are Alcoholics Anonymous and Narcotics Anonymous. These groups have chapters that meet in most areas. These groups follow a twelve-step program that holds participants accountable for their behavior. By supporting one another and working through the steps, addicts can regain control of their lives.

Addictions affect the entire family. They change the way family members interact with one another. Groups such as Co-Dependents Anonymous, Adult Children of Alcoholics, and Alateen are designed to help family members of people with addictions. They teach the family better ways to interact with the addict. In these groups, family members can meet others who are facing the same crisis. They can provide support and advice for each other.

Counselors, social workers, police officers, teachers, and religious leaders can often direct people to the help they need. These professionals may know about groups and agencies in the community. The Yellow Pages of many phone books also provide contact information about these groups and agencies.

Responding to Crises

What happens to someone who is involved in a crisis? How does this person respond? The answer to these questions will vary widely. A person's response to crisis depends on many factors. Some of these are listed in Figure 10-10. What other factors can you identify?

Factors That Influence Crisis Effects
- how serious the crisis was
- how long the crisis lasted
- whether the crisis was expected or unexpected
- whether trauma or injury was involved
- what other stress or crises the person was experiencing at the time
- what personal resources the person has to deal with the crisis
- how much crisis a person has faced in the past and how he or she has handled it
- what coping mechanisms the person learned from family
- how the crisis affected the person's loved ones
- what kind of support the person has

These factors may affect how a person will respond to crisis.

Facing a crisis can be difficult. It may involve many intense emotions that are tough to experience. It is important to work through crises, however. Ignoring them won't make them go away. Denying a problem exists will not solve it. Both ignoring and denying can cause many additional problems. These responses can also delay your recovery from the crisis. It is usually best to work through a crisis as soon as possible after it occurs.

Personal Resources

How you respond to crisis will depend largely on your personal resources. These are qualities you have that will help you meet needs and solve problems. Personal resources will help you deal with outside pressures. As a teen, it is worth while for you to develop mental resources. You will rely on them throughout your lifetime.

For instance, you might be a really strong person who bounces back easily. It's possible you might deny the effects of a crisis at the time but break down months later. You might be devastated when a crisis occurs but slowly work through your feelings and recover. Knowing which of these is your style will help you meet crises in the best way you can.

Other examples are patience, courage, a good attitude, spiritual beliefs, and self-esteem. Each of these personal resources will help you recover from crises. Being able to deal with stress and develop coping skills makes a big difference. Sharing your feelings with others and asking for support will also help.

Your attitude is a key personal resource. **Attitude** refers to your outlook about life in general or a specific situation. Your attitude toward what has happened will greatly affect how you react. If you have a negative attitude, you are likely to focus on the difficult or bad parts of life or a situation. You may feel things will never improve or you will never get over what happened. This will make it much harder for you to recover from crises. It will also make depression more likely.

A positive attitude will help you overcome hardship. By focusing on the good aspects of a situation, you can help yourself feel better. You can take a bad event and help yourself think differently about it. With a positive attitude, you believe things will work out for the best. In difficult times, you believe you will get through them and be okay in time.

How much courage you have also makes a difference. Courage will help you work through a crisis and resolve it. You may need courage to make changes. Courage allows you to face danger, change, or pain despite your fear. See Figure 10-11.

Sometimes you will need the courage to accept that a situation cannot be changed. When a person close to you dies, you can't bring the person back. It takes courage to let him or her go. When a child is born with disabilities, parents must accept her as she is. It takes courage to accept this, but with acceptance comes strength. This strength can help families continue after a crisis.

> **Craig's Example: Facing a Crisis with Courage**
>
> Craig's mom was an alcoholic. She would stay up late at night drinking and neglect her job and other responsibilities. Craig and his dad were worried about her. They were upset about how her drinking was affecting the family, too. They decided it would be best to have a family meeting and share their concern for her. Craig's dad called the local chapter of Alcoholics Anonymous for advice on how to best structure the meeting. After the meeting, Craig's mom checked herself into an alcohol rehabilitation program. Craig and his dad went for counseling. Craig was very thankful he and his dad had the courage to confront his mom. Craig's mom recovered from her addiction and their family life improved. Craig knew he would never regret his action, even though it had been a hard thing to do.

 In this case study, Craig and his dad need courage to face a family crisis.

For example, Colleen's baby sister was born with a disability. Her health care provider said she would never walk. The family grieved. They got support from their family, friends, and house of worship. As they began to accept her condition, they found the strength to face each day. Soon they were enjoying her wonderful personality.

How you manage your finances can be a personal resource. If you are financially prepared, you can keep unexpected expenses from turning into crises. You can do this by saving and buying insurance. Keeping your credit rating strong will allow you to borrow money if needed in a crisis.

Health can be a resource. Good health can help you meet crises with vigor and determination. Maintaining healthy habits helps you meet challenges you face. These habits include getting the right amounts of rest, activity, and nutritious food. Avoiding harmful substances will also improve your health.

Family Influences

Your response to crisis will also be influenced by what you saw modeled in the family you grew up in. If the adults reacted calmly and quickly to an emergency, you may react the same way. If they panicked when a crisis arose, you may be inclined to panic, too. Sometimes you may find that an example others set for you is ineffective. In this case, you can choose not to follow it. You've learned by example what doesn't work. This can help you as you face crises.

In times of crisis, families and friends also support each other. This support can have a tremendous effect on a person's ability to face crisis. Family members may provide emotional support by listening. They can remind the loved one they care with kind words, cards, flowers, or gifts. Emotional pain takes time to heal. It is important for friends and family to continue to show they care for several months after the crisis occurs.

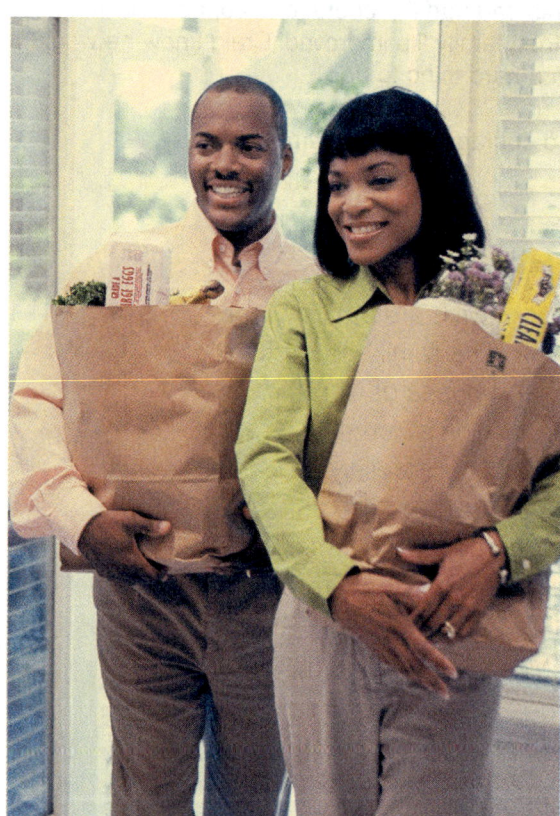

10-12 During a crisis, friends and family might help by running errands, such as shopping for groceries.

Families can also offer practical support, such as helping with meals, child care, housing, or household tasks. This kind of support can free the person to handle other matters or take some time alone. Sometimes family members can give financial help as well. Having whatever support friends and family can provide encourages a person to work through a crisis and heal. Friends and family often want to help in times like these. See Figure 10-12.

Jillian's best friend, Raquel, died in a car accident. Jillian knew Raquel's parents were devastated. She sent flowers soon after the accident. A few months later, she sent a card to let them know she cared. On Raquel's birthday, Jillian visited with Raquel's parents. They visited the gravesite together and shared stories about Raquel. Jillian asked how they were handling things. She encouraged them to talk with their minister about their pain. When Jillian went home, she knew she had helped, and this made her feel good about herself.

Community Resources

Even with all the resources within families, outside help is often needed in times of crisis. Some people feel seeking outside help is a sign of failure. This isn't true. In fact, identifying the help you need means you're taking care of yourself. Seeking that help is a sign you are trying to solve the problem. You can find help in many places within the community. The most common of these are social service agencies, support groups, religious groups, schools, and counselors.

Social Service Agencies

A social service agency is an agency within the community that exists to serve the public. The purpose of these agencies is to help people in need. Some of these agencies are funded by the government. Others are run by nonprofit or religious groups. You may be able to find these agencies listed in the phone book. You can also ask a teacher, school counselor, or other trusted adult to help you find them.

The services each agency provides will vary. This depends mostly on the crises each program is designed to assist with. Some offer emotional support through counseling. Others can give financial support. If the crisis involves a violent crime, a worker from a social service agency might accompany the victim to court.

Some social service agencies offer support groups. These groups offer a meeting place for people who share the same crisis. The best-known support group is Alcoholics Anonymous. In a support group, members talk about their concerns and ask advice from one another. They share their feelings and offer emotional support. Support groups can help a person feel less alone. Often, groups meet weekly and at little or no cost to the members. A support group may or may not be led by a worker from a social service agency.

Religious Groups

For some people, religious groups can be a valuable source of support. Spiritual beliefs help many people overcome crises in their lives. Coming together with other members at services and other events can bring a sense of comfort in troubled times. For some, other members can become like an extended family. These can be people to call when help is needed.

Members of a religious group can usually talk to their religious leader about crises that occur. These leaders often offer counseling to their members at no cost. They can advise members about faith issues and personal matters. A religious leader may be a source of support.

Some houses of worship also offer classes or seminars on key issues. Taking these classes may help people avoid or overcome a crisis. Some of the topics presented might include the following:

- financial planning
- parenting skills
- healthy relationships
- addictions
- stress management
- single parent issues
- grief

If you want to learn more, you can contact the house of worship that interests you. Ask what services are available. The services provided by a religious group may be valuable to you in everyday life as well as during crises.

School Resources

You may be able to find many of the resources you need through your school. In some schools, you can take classes in parenting skills, attend support groups, and get medical care for you and your child. Other schools don't provide as many of these services. In most schools, however, you can make an appointment to see a counselor or social worker. This person can talk to you about your concerns. He or she can refer you to any other services you might need. Teachers and advisers may also be able to assist you by listening or directing you to other resources. See Figure 10-13.

Counselors

In times of crisis, you might need to see a professional counselor. This type of counselor usually charges a fee. This fee may be based upon your ability to pay or covered by insurance. You can ask what the fees are before you schedule an appointment.

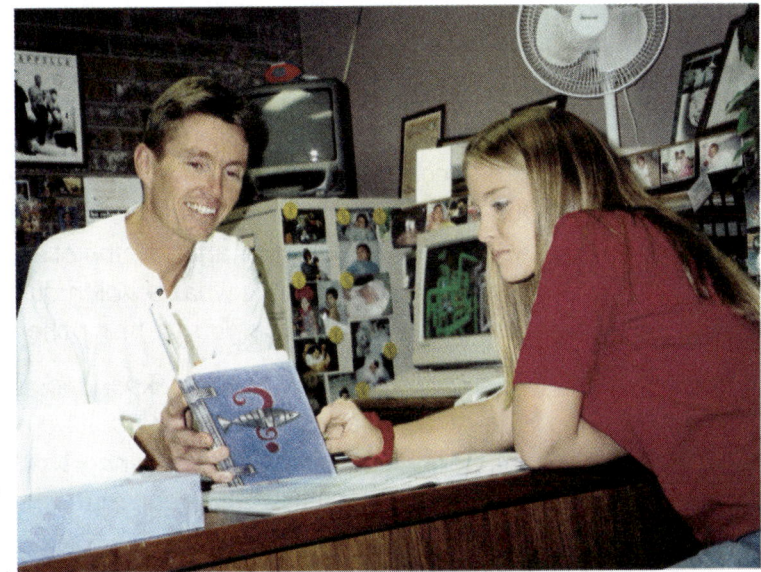

10-13 Your teacher, adviser, or counselor can help you find support, as well as many of the other resources you might need.

Some professional counselors specialize in one area. For example, an addictions counselor deals mainly with issues related to addiction. For help with other issues, you would need to seek help elsewhere. Other counselors see clients with a variety of concerns. This type of counselor may not know as much about a particular area of concern, however. As you look for a counselor, decide which type of counselor would best meet your needs.

Some counselors do individual counseling, while others prefer to work with the entire family. What affects one member affects them all. All of them must work together to overcome unhealthy attitudes and actions. Again, you will want to choose the type of counselor you think would best suit your needs.

Seeing a counselor can help you work through problems. It can help you resolve negative feelings related to a crisis. Exploring these painful issues isn't easy, though. It takes time to heal from the pain and overcome the crisis. By having the courage to face these issues, you are taking a giant step toward recovery.

Nonhuman Resources

Using human resources can be a great way to handle your concerns. You can also solve problems by using nonhuman resources. For instance, you can use the library or the Internet to learn more about problems you face. Read books, magazines, newspapers, encyclopedias, brochures, and pamphlets. This can help you find some solutions. Understanding what's going on can also boost your confidence and motivate you to find other help you may need.

Major Points

- Everyone will experience some crises in life. Some crises surround positive changes. Others are the result of bad things that have happened. You, your family, and your relationships will face crises from time to time.

- Depression is common among teens. It can be the result of other crises or a crisis on its own. Severe cases of depression can lead people to consider suicide. For this reason, it's important to seek help if you or someone you know is depressed.

- Domestic violence is any action meant to hurt a family member or dating partner. Forms include neglect and physical, emotional, and sexual abuse. Over time, violence often gets worse. Ending the abuse often means leaving the relationship.

- Being the victim of a sexual crime is traumatic. It can take a long time for victims to recover from this crisis. Although reporting the incident is difficult, it's important. This will allow the victim to get help and the police to catch the perpetrator.

- Substance abuse and addiction can have severe consequences for an individual. They can also result in crisis for the entire family and other loved ones. Ending substance abuse may involve medical treatment, counseling, and support groups.

- Each person responds to crisis in a unique way. This depends on a number of factors. The personal resources, family influences, and community resources a person has can make a big difference in his or her response to crisis.

Glossary

A

abortion. The removal of an embryo or fetus from the uterus before birth to end a pregnancy. (6)

abstinence. Choosing to postpone having sex until a time in life when you're ready to enter this type of relationship. (8)

abuser. The person in a violent relationship who hurts one or more loved ones. (10)

accommodate. Choosing to go along with another person's wishes instead of your own to resolve a conflict. (9)

acquired immunodeficiency syndrome (AIDS). A deadly disease of the immune system caused by a virus called HIV. (8)

active listening. Type of listening in which the listener focuses on the message and shows he or she understands it. (9)

addiction. Dependence of the mind or body upon a substance. (10)

adoption. The legal process of transferring parenting rights and responsibilities from a child's birthparents to adoptive parents. (6)

adoption agency. An organization that has been licensed by the state to help people plan adoptions. (6)

adoptive parent. A person who becomes a parent through the adoption of a child. (5)

aggressive behavior. Behavior that violates the rights of others in an attempt to get your own way. (9)

assertive behavior. Behavior that allows you to express your feelings and needs directly. (9)

attitude. Your outlook on life in general or about a specific situation. (10)

B

baby blues. Name for moderately depressed feelings a woman may experience for a short time after giving birth. (10)

babysitter. Person who is paid to provide child care for a few hours at a time. (7)

belittling. Actions or comments that cause someone to seem or feel less of a person. (10)

biological parent. A person who becomes a parent through the birth of his or her child; birthparent. (5)

birth control pill. Daily hormone pill that prevents pregnancy by keeping a woman's body from releasing an egg. (8)

birthparent. A person who becomes a parent through the birth of his or her child; biological parent. (5)

boundary. Physical, emotional, or mental limit a person sets for his or her behavior and what behavior he or she will accept from others. (8)

budget. Personal spending plan. (7)

C

cervical cap. Thimble-shaped rubber or plastic cap that firmly covers the opening of the cervix to prevent sperm from meeting the egg; used to prevent pregnancy. (8)

cervical shield. A dome-shaped rubber or plastic barrier that has an air valve and loop to aid in removal that firmly covers the opening of the cervix to prevent sperm from meeting the egg; used to prevent pregnancy. (8)

chancre. Sore that appears during the first stage of syphilis at the site where the person was infected. (8)

child abuse. Any abuse in which the victim is younger than 18 years of age. (10)

child care provider. Person whose job is to take care of children on a regular basis for an extended period of time, such as daily. (7)

chlamydia. The most common STI among teens; it is caused by bacteria and can be cured with antibiotics. (8)

closed adoption. Type of adoption in which there is no contact between the birthparents and the adoptive family. (6)

collaboration. Way to resolve a conflict in which everyone involved works together to find a solution that is acceptable to all. (9)

communication skills. The skills a person needs to understand others and help others understand him or her. (1)

community resources. Facilities and services a person can access just by being part of a community. (3)

compromise. Way to resolve a conflict in which each person gives up a little of what he or she wanted in order to reach a middle ground. (9)

conditional love. A type of love that is given only when certain conditions are met; love with limits. (5)

condom. A thin sheath that fits over the erect penis to keep semen from entering a woman's body during sex; used to prevent pregnancy and protect against STIs. (8)

congenital disorder. A health problem or condition that is inherited and present from birth. (5)

consequences. Possible results of a decision; can be positive or negative. (3)

constructive resolution. A resolution in which everyone is satisfied with the results and the relationship is preserved. (9)

contraceptive. Any method a couple uses to keep the woman from conceiving. (8)

contraceptive injection. A contraceptive injection that contains a synthetic hormone that prevents a woman's egg cells from being released. (8)

contraceptive sponge. Small round polyurethane sponge that is placed inside the woman's vagina against the cervix to prevent pregnancy. (8)

co-parenting. Describes two parents who work together to raise their child although they are not married or in a romantic relationship. (5)

crab lice. Another name for pubic lice. (8)

crisis. A situation that causes distress and interrupts a person's normal way of thinking and coping. (10)

D

daily hassles. Little annoyances and stresses you face from day to day; one kind of stressor. (7)

date rape. Type of rape that occurs between people who are dating or did date in the past. (10)

decision-making process. Step-by-step process that can be used to make a decision. (1)

degrade. To attack a person's self-esteem through actions or words. (9)

depression. A lasting feeling of sadness and hopelessness. (10)

destructive resolution. Resolution in which feelings are hurt, negative emotions are experienced, and the relationship is damaged. (9)

diaphragm. A thin rubber cup with a rigid rim that covers the woman's cervix and keeps sperm from reaching the egg; used to prevent pregnancy. (8)

dishonesty. Showing a lack of truthfulness. (9)

distress. Negative type of stress. (7)

domestic violence. Any behavior that is meant to hurt a family member or dating partner. (10)

dual-career family. Family in which both parents work outside the home. (4)

E

emotional abuse. Abuse that hurts a person's feelings or self-esteem. (10)

emotional boundary. Limits a person sets on allowing others to manipulate him or her and play on his or her emotions. (8)

empathy. The ability to see a situation from someone else's point of view; being able to relate to a person's feelings without having those same feelings yourself. (9)

F

feedback. Letting someone know how you felt about what he or she said to you. (9)

female condom. Polyurethane sheath that fits inside a woman's vagina to catch sperm and keep them from entering a woman's body; used to prevent pregnancy. (8)

fight. To try to win a conflict by either verbal or physical means. (1)

fight or flight response. The body's natural response that occurs as an attempt to either fight off the cause of stress or escape from it. (7)

final adoption hearing. Court hearing that occurs after a child has been placed with the adoptive parents; time when the court declares the adoption final and legal. (6)

flee. To run away from, avoid, or ignore a conflict. (1)

foster parent. An adult who serves as a parent by volunteering to provide a temporary home to a child in need of one. (5)

G

genital herpes. A serious, incurable STI that is caused by the herpes simplex virus; includes breakouts of blisters that occur from time to time throughout life. (8)

genital warts. Incurable STI that includes small, hard growths in the reproductive organs, bladder, and rectum; caused by the human papilloma virus (HPV). (8)

goal. A statement of something a person wants to accomplish. (3)

gonorrhea. Common STI that is caused by bacteria, often has no symptoms, and can be cured with antibiotics. (8)

H

hepatitis type B. A serious virus that causes liver damage and liver cancer and can be spread sexually. (8)

herpes simplex virus (HSV). Virus that causes genital herpes; spread by sexual contact with an infected person. (8)

home study. Visit to the home of people who wish to adopt by an adoption agency before the adoption takes place; done to ensure the home is safe and adequate for a child. (6)

hormone. Chemical that controls or affects one of your body systems. (1)

Glossary

human immunodeficiency virus (HIV). Virus that breaks down the immune system and eventually leads to AIDS; can be transmitted sexually. (8)

human papilloma virus (HPV). Virus that causes genital warts; often spread through sexual contact. (8)

human resources. Resources that come from within a person. (3)

hygiene. Habits of maintaining personal cleanliness. (4)

I

I-message. A statement that focuses on the speaker's feelings and most often begins with the word I. (9)

immune system. The body system that fights disease. (7)

impulsive. Acting without thinking beforehand about the consequences. (10)

incest. Any sexual activity that occurs between family members other than spouses. (10)

independent adoptions. Type of adoption that is not arranged through a state-licensed adoption agency. (6)

independent adoption service. An organization that works with adoption but is not licensed by the state. (6)

infatuation. An intense feeling of attraction that begins quickly and fades over time. (4)

instinctive. Based on a natural skill or ability rather than being taught or learned. (5)

intrauterine device (IUD). Small, flexible plastic device that is inserted by a health care provider into the woman's uterus to prevent pregnancy for a period of one to eight years; not recommended for use by teens. (8)

L

long-term goal. A plan to accomplish something within a relatively long period of time; usually more than a year. (3)

love. A strong, steady, and long-lasting feeling of attachment, warmth, and understanding between two people that builds slowly over time. (4)

M

major life event. A happening that brings great change into your life; one type of stressor. (7)

mandated reporter. Professional, such as a teacher or health care provider, who is required by law to report known or suspected cases of child abuse to the authorities. (10)

marital rape. Type of rape that occurs between spouses. (10)

marriage. The emotional and legal commitment a man and woman make to become husband and wife. (4)

material resources. Type of resources that includes money and all the items a person owns. (3)

mental boundary. Limit a person sets to protect his or her own thoughts and beliefs rather than being swayed by others. (8)

mifepristone. Prescription medicine given by a health care provider to induce an abortion by blocking a hormone that sustains the pregnancy. (6)

N

National Adoption Information Clearinghouse. A national agency that provides adoption information sheets to the public; has current information on each state's adoption laws. (6)

natural family planning. Contraceptive method in which a couple tries to predict a woman's most fertile days and abstain from sex during these days; not recommended for use by teens. (8)

neglect. Holding back or failing to provide something that is needed; a type of domestic violence. (10)

nonverbal communication. The use of a message that doesn't require words; includes posture, body language, gestures, tone of voice, and facial expressions. (9)

O

open adoption. Type of adoption in which there is some type of contact between the adoptive family and the birthparents during or after the adoption. (6)

openness. Describes how much contact the birthparents have with the adoptive family during and after an adoption. (6)

order of protection. A court order that sets clear terms to protect a victim from further domestic violence. (10)

P

passive behavior. Behavior that allows others to do what they want, in spite of how you feel. (9)

paternity. Biological fatherhood of a child; can be admitted voluntarily or proven though the court with DNA testing. (5)

perpetrator. Person who commits a crime. (10)

personal resources. The qualities you have that will help you meet needs and solve problems. (10)

physical abuse. Injuries someone purposely causes to another person's body. (10)

physical boundary. Limit placed on where and how a person wants to touch another person and be touched by him or her. (8)

postpartum depression. Extreme and lasting feelings of depression some women experience following the birth of a child. (10)

Glossary

prejudice. An unfair opinion or judgment made about people of another group without first getting to know them. (9)

prenatal care. Medical care that is given during pregnancy. (1)

prioritize. To decide which things are most important to you; to set priorities. (3)

private adoption agency. Type of adoption agency that is run by a private group instead of by the government; most common type of agency used by teen birthparents. (6)

provider. Traditional marital role for a man that included earning a living, making decisions for the family, and managing the finances. (4)

pubic lice. Tiny gray parasites that attach to the hair of the pubic area, are very contagious, and can be passed by close physical contact, including sex; also called crab lice. (8)

public adoption agency. Type of adoption agency that is run by the state government to place children who are in the custody of the state into adoptive homes. (6)

put-down. A comment meant to make the other person look bad in an attempt to make yourself look good. (9)

R

rape. Forcing a person to have sexual intercourse without his or her consent. (10)

residential parent. Parent with whom a child lives if both parents do not live together with the child. (5)

resolve. To work with another person to settle a conflict in a way that satisfies both people. (1)

resources. The means a person has for reaching goals. (3)

role. A set of behaviors that is linked to a certain position a person fills in life. (4)

S

scabies. A skin infection that is caused by mites and can be spread by close physical or sexual contact. (8)

secondary virginity. Name sometimes given to the decision to practice abstinence after having sex in the past. (8)

self-control. The ability to monitor your own actions and make appropriate choices. (7)

self-esteem. The amount of confidence and satisfaction a person has with himself or herself as a person. (1)

self-pity. Feeling sorry for yourself. (10)

self-talk. The messages you send yourself about you; can be positive or negative. (2)

sexual abuse. Type of domestic violence that involves sexual activity or issues. (10)

sexual assault. Any kind of forced sexual behavior. (10)

sexually transmitted disease (STD). A name sometimes used to describe an STIs. (8)

sexually transmitted infection (STI). An infection spread from person to person through sexual contact. (8)

short-term goal. A plan to accomplish something within a relatively short period of time; often within a week, month, or year. (3)

shotgun wedding. Phrase used to describe forced marriages that were once common among pregnant teens and their partners. (4)

sibling rivalry. Strong competitive and jealous feelings between brothers and sisters; especially common when children are spaced close together. (8)

single parenting. Type of parenting in which one parent raises a child on his or her own and has full responsibility for the child's care. (5)

skin patch. A contraceptive device that looks like a bandage that a woman attaches to her lower stomach, buttocks, or upper body. It releases hormones into the bloodstream that can prevent pregnancy. (8)

spermicide. A chemical used in foams, creams, jellies, films, and tablets to prevent pregnancy by killing sperm or making them unable to swim toward an egg. (8)

stepparent. A person who becomes a parent through marriage. (5)

sterility. Permanent loss of the ability to have a child biologically. (6)

sterilization. The use of surgery to prevent conception permanently. (8)

stress. The tension you feel as a response to change. (7)

stressor. A source of stress. (7)

substance abuse. Allowing the use of a substance to interfere with your life. (10)

suicide. The act of taking one's own life. (10)

supporter. Traditional marital role for a woman that included caring for and maintaining the home as well as raising the children. (4)

support group. A group of people who meet to discuss a challenge or concern they have in common. (2)

support system. The network of people and organizations you can rely upon in times of need. (2)

sympathy. The act of sharing another person's feelings. (9)

syphilis. A three-stage STI that is caused by bacteria and can be cured with penicillin; effects become more serious in each stage. (8)

T

trichomoniasis (trich). An infection that is caused by a one-celled animal called a protozoan and is often spread sexually. (8)

trust. A feeling of being able to believe in and rely on someone. (9)

tubal ligation. Sterilization surgery of a female that permanently blocks her fallopian tubes so eggs cannot travel to the uterus to be fertilized. (8)

U

unconditional love. Type of love that does not have conditions or limits; the type of love children need from their parents. (5)

V

vacuum aspiration. Medical procedure used to perform an abortion in which a suction tube is placed into the uterus to remove its contents. (6)

vaginal contraceptive ring. A flexible, transparent ring that is placed in the vagina where it releases hormones that prevent the egg from being fertilized. (8)

vaginal infections. Infections caused by the overgrowth of bacteria, causing the vagina to become infected, swell, itch, and have a discharge. (8)

value conflict. Tension that occurs when two values or sets of values disagree. (3)

values. Your beliefs, feelings, and ideas about what is important. (3)

vasectomy. Sterilization surgery of a male that blocks his vas deferens so sperm cannot travel through them to be released. (8)

verbal communication. The use of words to send or receive a message. (9)

victim. Person who has been hurt by domestic violence, sexual assault, rape, incest, or another crime. (10)

visualize. To form an image in one's mind, usually of success, such as meeting a goal. (2)

W

withdrawal. Symptoms an addict experiences as his or her body rids itself of the drug to which it's addicted. (10)

Y

yeast infection. Most common kind of vaginal infection; caused by an overgrowth of bacteria in the vagina. (8)

you-message. Message that focuses on the listener's role in a problem and begins with the word _you_. (9)

Index

A

Abortion, 116-120
  definition, 116
  emotional issues, 118
  future effects, 120
  medical issues, 117, 118
  personal beliefs, 118
  social issues, 118
  support, 119
Abstinence, 166, 167
Abusive relationships,
    see <u>Domestic violence</u>.
Abuser, 219-225
Accommodate, 208, 209
Acquired immunodeficiency syndrome
    (AIDS), 169, 170
Active listening, 192-196
Addiction, 231, 232
Adjusting to parenting, 126-155
  comparing roles, 126-128
  demands, 128-138
  finding a babysitter, 137, 138
  money management, 131, 132
  part-time job, 135-137
  relationships, 138-149
  schoolwork management, 133-135
  time management, 129-131
Adoption, 107-116
  agencies, 108-110
  closed, 112
  definition, 107
  feelings about, 114-116
  home study, 110
  independent, 110-112
  openness, 112, 113
  process, 114
  reasons, 113, 114
Adoption agency, 108-110
Adoptive parent, 89, 107-116
Aggressive behavior, 199, 200
AIDS, 169, 170
Anger, handling, 198, 199
Assertive behavior, 199, 200
Attitude, 234

B

Baby blues, 216
Babysitter, 137, 138
Belittling, 222
Biological parent, 89
Birth control, see <u>Contraceptives</u>.
Birth control pill, 181, 182
Birthparent, 89, 107-116
Blaming 48, 49, 123, 201
Boundary, 158
Budget, 132

Index

C

Careers, see <u>Work</u>.
Cervical cap, 186
Cervical shield, 186
Chancre, 173
Child abuse, 221-224
Child care provider, 137
Child's needs, 32, 95-96
Child support, 143
Chlamydia, 170
Closed adoption, 112
Collaboration, 209
Communication,
  barriers, 201, 202
  being assertive, 199, 200
  conflicts, 207-211
  controlling emotions, 193, 194
  effective speaking, 196
  elements, 191-200
  empathy, 195
  eye contact, 193, 203, 204
  handling anger, 198, 199
  relationships, 190-211
  skills, 30
  types, 191, 192
  with children, 203, 204
  with co-parent, 204, 205
  with parents, 206
Community resources, 59, 60, 237-239
Compromise, 209
Conditional love, 95, 96
Condoms, 184, 185
Conflict, 207-211
  causes of, 207, 208
  outcomes, 208
  resolution, 30, 31, 209-211
    options, 30, 31
    steps, 209-211
  ways to handle, 208, 209

Congenital disorder, 93
Consequences, 65, 66, 121, 122
Constructive resolution, 208
Contraceptive injection, 182
Contraceptives, 180-188
  abstinence, 181
  birth control pill, 181, 182
  cervical cap, 186
  cervical shield, 186
  condoms, 184-185
  contraceptive injection, 182
  contraceptive sponge, 186
  deciding about, 188
  definition, 180
  diaphragm, 185
  IUD, 187
  methods, 180-187
  natural family planning, 186, 187
  skin patch, 182
  spermicide, 183, 184
  sterilization, 187
  vaginal contraceptive ring, 183
Contraceptive sponge, 186
Co-parenting, 99, 100, 142-146
Crab lice, 175, 176
Crisis,
  addiction, 231, 232
  child abuse, 221-224
  common, 214-232
  community resources, 237-239
  definition, 213
  depression, 215-219
  domestic violence, 219-226
  family influences, 235, 236
  incest, 226-231
  in relationships, 213-240
  rape, 226-231
  sexual assault, 226-231
  substance abuse, 231, 232
  suicide, 217-219

D

Dads, young, see Fathers, young.
Daily hassles, 150
Date rape, 227, 229
Decision-making process, 29, 62-68, 120-123
  choosing best option, 66, 67, 122
  consequences, 65, 66, 121, 122
  definition, 29
  evaluating options, 65, 66, 121, 122
  evaluating results, 67, 68, 122, 123
  examining information, 120, 121
  gathering information, 120, 121
  identifying decision, 62, 63, 120
  identifying options, 65, 121
Decisions,
  abortion, 116-120
  adoption, 107-116
  contraceptives, 188
  parenting, 105-107
  pregnancy-related, 28, 29, 120-123
  self-esteem and, 37
  sexual, 156-188
Degrade, 197
Depression, 215-219
Destructive resolution, 208
Diaper bag, 129
Diaphragm, 185
Dishonesty, 201
Distress, 149
Domestic violence, 219-226
  abusers, 219-226
  definition, 219
  forms of abuse, 221, 222
  seeking help, 223-226
  steps to prevent, 225
  victims, 219-226
Dual-career family, 78, 79

E

Education, importance of, 20, 21, 36, 37, 133-135
Emotional abuse, 222
Emotional boundary, 158
Emotional needs of children, 32
Empathy, 195
Employment, see Work.

F

Family relationships, 18, 19, 52, 139-142, 235, 237
Family planning, see Contraceptives.
Fathers, young, 14, 18, 25, 81-87, 89-103, 105-107, 119, 142-146, 204, 205
Feedback, 196
Female condom, 185
Fight, 31
Fight or flight response, 151
Final adoption hearing, 114
Financial support, 78, 79, 84, 91, 92, 95, 97-103, 106, 131, 132, 135-137, 142, 143, 150, 180
Flee, 31
Foster parent, 89
Friends, 19, 52, 53, 147, 149

G

Genital herpes, 171, 172
Genital warts, 172
Goals, 20-23, 57-62
  and resources, 58-60
  and values, 58
  definition, 57
  effects of pregnancy, 20-23
  setting, 60-62
  specific, 61
Gonorrhea, 171

Index

H
Hepatitis type B, 173, 174
Herpes simplex virus (HSV), 171, 172
HIV, 169, 170
Home study, 110
Hormone, 17
HPV, 172
HSV, 171, 172
Human immunodeficiency virus (HIV), 169, 170
Human papilloma virus (HPV), 172
Human resources, 58, 59
Hygiene, 82, 83

I
I-message, 197, 201, 206
Immune system, 151
Incest, 229-231
Independent adoption, 110-112
Independent adoption service, 111
Infatuation, 69, 70
Instinctive, 89, 90
Intellectual needs of children, 32
Intrauterine device, 187
IUD, 187

J
Job, 21, 22, 36, 37, 78, 79, 94, 95, 135-137
  dual-career family, 78, 79
  parenting decisions and, 94, 95
  performance and self-esteem, 36, 37
  pregnancy and, 21, 22
  safety during pregnancy, 22
  schedules, co-parents, 99
  single parenting and, 103
  stress and, 150
  teen parents, part-time, 135-137

L
Listening, active 192, 193
Long-term goal, 57
Love, 69-71

M
Major life event, 149
Managing money, 131, 132
Managing time, 129-131
Mandated reporters, 223
Marital rape, 227
Marriages, teen, 69-87
  adjustment, 79, 80
  definition, 69
  deciding about, 80-87
  failure, 76, 77
  infatuation and, 69-71
  love and, 69-71
  pregnancy and, 71, 72
  readiness, 84, 85
  reasons, 69-75
  roles, 78, 79
  waiting, 85, 87
Material resources, 59
Media influences, 53
Mental boundary, 158
Mifepristone, 118
Mutual, 75

N
National Adoption Information Clearinghouse, 108
Natural family planning, 186, 187
Negative self-talk, 43, 45
Neglect, 222
Nonhuman resources, 240
Nonverbal communication, 191

O

Open adoption, 112
Openness in adoption, 112, 113
Order of protection, 223

P

Parents,
  adoptive, 89, 107-116
  biological, 89
  birthparents, 89, 107-116
  foster, 89
  married teen, 75, 79, 80, 94, 98
  of teens, 18, 19, 24, 25, 33, 39, 40, 51, 52, 72, 74, 139-142
  residential, 99
  roles of, 126-128
  single, 102-104
  stepparents, 89
Parenting, teen, 89-107, 126-155
  adjusting to, 126-155
  deciding about, 91-97
    abilities needed, 95, 96
    age, 94
    career factors, 94, 95
    feelings, 95
    finances, 95
    health, 93
    relationship stability, 94
    work factors, 94, 95
  options, 97-104
    co-parents, 99, 100
    marriage, 98
    supportive family, 100, 101
  readiness, 96, 97
  reasons, 91-93
  responsibilities, 90
  rewards, 90
  roles, 89-91
  self-esteem and, 38, 39
  single parenting, 102-104
  with family support, 100, 101
  within marriage, 98
Partner relationship, 18, 146, 147
Passive behavior, 199
Paternity, 103
Perpetrator, 226
Personal resources, 233-235
Physical abuse, 221
Physical boundary, 158
Physical needs of children, 32
Positive self-talk, 43, 45
Postpartum depression, 216
Pregnancy, teen, 14-33
  accepting, 15-23
  changes, 16-23
    emotional, 16-18
    goals, 20-23
    physical, 16, 17
    plans, 20-23
    relationships, 18, 19
  child's needs, 31, 32
  coping, 32, 33
  decisions about, 105-123
  handling news of, 15, 16
  options, 105-124
  preventing repeat, 178-188
  telling others, 24-28
    negative reactions, 26-28
    right time, 24, 25
    right way, 25, 26
Prejudice, 202
Prenatal care, 16, 17
Prioritize, 56
Private adoption agencies, 109, 110
Provider, 78
Pubic lice, 175, 176
Public adoption agencies, 109, 110
Put-down, 202

Index

R

Rape, 222, 226-231
Relationships, 156-188
  building, 156-160
  changing expectations in, 138, 149
  communicating, 190-211
  co-parent, 99, 100, 142-146
  crises in, 213-240
  healthy, 31, 156-158
  partner, 18, 146-147
  unhealthy, 158-160
Religious influences, 53
Repeat pregnancy, 178-188
Residential parent, 99
Resolve, 31
Resources, 58-60
Responsibility, 48, 49, 123
Role, 78, 126-128

S

Scabies, 176
School, 20, 21, 36, 37, 54, 133-135
Secondary virginity, 181
Self-control, 132
Self-esteem, 34-49
  decision making and, 37
  definition, 29
  evaluating, 42-44
  formation, 39-42
  goals and, 36, 37
  health and, 36
  importance, 35-39
  improving, 43-49
  parenting and, 38, 39
  performance and, 36, 37
  personal care and, 36
  personal outlook and, 35
  relationships and, 38
Self-pity, 217
Self-talk, 43, 45
Sexual abuse, 222
Sexual assault, 226-231
Sexual decisions, 160-167
  abstinence, 166-167
  contraception, 178-188
  factors, 162-166
  STIs, 167-178
Sexually transmitted disease, 167
Sexually transmitted infections, 167-178
  definition, 167
  prevention, 167-178
  reducing risks, 168
  treating, 176-178
  types, 169-178
Short-term goal, 57
Shotgun weddings, 72
Sibling rivalry, 180
Single parenting, 102-104
Skin patch, 182
Social needs of children, 32
Speaking, effective, 196, 197
Spermicide, 183, 184
Stepparent, 89
Sterility, 117
Sterilization, 187
STI, 167
  treatment, 176-178
Stress,
  causes of, 149-151
  dealing with, 149-155
  definition, 149
  effects, 151, 152
  preventing, 154, 155
  reducing, 153, 154
Stressor, 149
Substance abuse, 231, 232
Suicide, 217-219

Supporter, 78
Support group, 48
Support system, 47
Sympathy, 195
Syphilis, 172, 173

T

Teen fathers, see Fathers, young.
Teen marriage, see Marriages, teen.
Teen parenting, see Parenting, teen.
Teen pregnancy, see Pregnancy, teen.
Teen roles, 126-128
Trichomoniasis, 174, 175
Trust, 201, 204
Tubal ligation, 187

U

Unconditional love, 95

V

Vacuum aspiration, 117
Vaginal contraceptive ring, 183
Vaginal infections, 176
Value conflict, 55, 56
Values, 50-57, 162
  changing, 56, 57
  conflict, 55, 56
  definition, 50
  development, 51-54
  influences, 51-54
  sexual decisions and, 162, 163
Vasectomy, 187
Verbal communication, 191
Victim, 219-225
Visualize, 46

W

Withdrawal, 232
Work, 21, 22, 36, 37, 78, 79, 94, 95, 135-137
  dual-career family, 78, 79
  parenting decisions and, 94, 95
  performance and self-esteem, 36, 37
  pregnancy and, 21, 22
  safety during pregnancy, 22
  schedules, co-parents, 99
  single parenting and, 103
  stress and, 150
  teen parents, part-time, 135-137

Y

Yeast infection, 176
You-messages, 197, 201